OSCEs for MRCOG Part 2

OSCEs for MRCOG Part 2
A self-assessment guide

Antony Hollingworth
Consultant in Obstetrics & Gynaecology, Whipps Cross University Hospital Trust; and Honorary Senior Lecturer at Queen Mary and Westfield College, London, UK

Janice Rymer
Professor in Obstetrics & Gynaecology at Guy's & St Thomas' NHS Foundation Trust, London; and Senior Lecturer at Guy's, King's and St Thomas' School of Medicine, London, UK

Hodder Arnold
A MEMBER OF THE HODDER HEADLINE GROUP

First published in Great Britain in 2005 by
Hodder Education, a member of the Hodder Headline Group,
338 Euston Road, London NW1 3BH

http://www.hoddereducation.com

Distributed in the United States of America by
Oxford University Press Inc.,
198 Madison Avenue, New York, NY10016
Oxford is a registered trademark of Oxford University Press

British Library Cataloguing in Publication Data
A catalogue record for this book is available from the British Library

Library of Congress Cataloging-in-Publication Data
A catalog record for this book is available from the Library of Congress

ISBN-10 0 340 814950
ISBN-13 978 0 340 814 950

1 2 3 4 5 6 7 8 9 10

Commissioning Editor: Sarah Burrows
Project Editor: Naomi Wilkinson
Production Controller: Joanna Walker
Cover Design: Georgina Hewitt
Index: Indexing Specialists (UK) Ltd

Typeset in 10 on 12pt Minion by Phoenix Photosetting, Lordwood, Chatham, Kent
Printed and bound in Malta

Dedication

This book is dedicated to our support systems: Ann, Roger, Victoria, Chloe and Adam

Contents

CONTENTS

Foreword

Achieving success in the MRCOG marks the beginning of joining a profession in which there must be continued professional development and learning. It is a hurdle to be conquered. Knowledge is not enough, technique is important.

The authors, Antony Hollingworth and Janice Rymer, are respected and experienced examiners used to setting marking schemes for the OSCE. This work will be an invaluable aid to study and self assessment. The scenarios used are all comparable to those met in the exam, and the properly prepared candidate would be well advised to consider using this book.

Roger Baldwin

Preface

The examination for the membership for the Royal College of Obstetricians and Gynaecologists aims to set a standard of competent, safe practice for anyone pursuing a career in obstetrics and gynaecology. The oral part of the examination now consists of Objective Structured Clinical Examinations (OSCEs). We have both been past or current chairman of the RCOG OSCE Committee, and convenors of the RCOG and Whipps Cross Hospital MRCOG courses. We therefore have extensive experience in teaching and preparing candidates for this examination, and also in examining candidates. In this book we have tried to give comprehensive examples of the type of OSCEs that you may come across and advice on how to approach these stations and the common problems that we have seen candidates encounter.

Remember that the written part of the examination concentrates on your knowledge, and the OSCEs will assess your application of knowledge, and skills. In our specialty, communication skills are especially important and we would hope that by going through this book and practising the OSCEs stations you will be competent in all the skills that the Royal College of Obstetricians and Gynaecologists expect you to have. We hope that you find this book invaluable in your preparation for the examination and we wish you luck.

Janice Rymer and Tony Hollingworth

Acknowledgements

We would like to thank the post graduate and examination departments at the Royal College of Obstetricians and Gynaecologists for their help and advice with the regulations and questions for the Part II MRCOG Examination.

We would also like to thank Naomi and Sarah at Hodder for their patience and encouragement at bringing this project to a timely delivery.

We would also like to acknowledge the influence of Roger Baldwin not only on our approach to learning and teaching but on many others who attended the Whipps Cross MRCOG course over the years. We would like to thank him for writing the foreword to this book.

Abbreviations

CDH	congenital dislocation of the hip
CRP	C-reactive protein
CTG	cardiotocograph
DVT	deep vein thrombosis
IDDM	insulin dependent diabetes mellitus
MDT	multi-disciplinary team
MRI	magnetic resonance imaging
NTD	neural tube defect
SCBU	special care baby unit
TAH	total abdominal hysterectomy
TED	thromboembolic deterant
TOP	termination of pregnancy
TPR	temperature, pulse and respiratory rate

Introduction

In the MRCOG Part II examination, knowledge is tested in the written paper by multiple choice questions and short essays. Clinical skills are tested in an objective structured clinical examination (OSCE) which replaces the traditional clinical long case and viva voce. The OSCE is designed to produce a valid and reproducible assessment of your skills. The MRCOG is a licensing examination and therefore the examination is not norm-referenced but criterion-referenced. This means that the minimum standard acceptable is decided before the test and you either reach that standard and pass, or you go below it and fail. This is much fairer than a norm-referenced examination where you may be disadvantaged if you go through with an experienced cohort of students or, likewise, you may be advantaged if you go through with a less experienced cohort.

Each candidate is exposed to the same set of scenarios. This means that the examination is reproducible and the marking is standardized. As you are exposed to 10 examiners, this improves the reliability of the examination.

The MRCOG Part II OSCE is a series of examinations based on clinical skills applied in a range of contexts where there is wide sampling with structured assessment and this improves the reliability. The OSCE currently consists of 10 marked stations and two preparatory stations. Each station lasts 15 minutes, and the duration of the examination is 3 hours. One minute before the conclusion of the station (at 14 minutes) there will be a bell to conclude the station and to allow the examiner to mark it. When this bell goes, move to the next station and read the relevant information. All the information relating to the station will be posted outside it as well as on the desk at the station. Take as much time as you need to read the information. You need to ensure you have read the question thoroughly; once you have grasped it, proceed into the station. This may take a few minutes but you are in control of your time. Do not be rushed. If you have just had a difficult station, you may need an extra minute or two to recover. As the information will be outside the station, this means that you will be in control of your timing. If you need the time, take it and make sure that you are calm and composed before you enter the next station.

This is a professional examination and respect for patients is important. You must dress appropriately and be well groomed. You must be polite and friendly and must transmit an air of confidence and competence to both the role-players and the examiners.

At the stations where there are patients, introduce yourself by your full name (first name only is too casual) and do your normal greeting (this may involve a handshake). Speak slowly and clearly and make eye contact. As you would normally do, observe their body language, as the role-players may have been instructed to behave in a certain way.

Of the 10 stations where an examiner is present, the candidate has to perform a task and each task tests knowledge, skills, communication or problem-solving abilities. Depending on the type of station there may be a role-player, a patient, some form of imaging, a pelvic model or a clinical scenario. As the examination evolves, new types of stations will be brought in. Currently the examination may include the following areas.

History-taking

This is a core skill and is included in every examination. Each candidate should be able to score very highly, but surprisingly the marks for this type of station are consistently low. It is important to take a comprehensive history, not only of the presenting complaint but of all the past histories. One logical approach is to ask an open-ended question about the patient's presentation and then comprehensively go through the presenting complaint; then go to past obstetric and gynaecology history and with the previous pregnancies note whether there were any problems, whether they were induced or spontaneous labour, whether there was a normal delivery and whether there were any intrapartum and/or postpartum problems. The weight and sex of the babies should be recorded. If there are any miscarriages or terminations, it is important to know whether evacuations were performed and whether there were any postoperative problems. A functional enquiry of all the systems should be undertaken, followed by medication history (which includes alcohol and recreational drug use), known allergies, family history and social history.

One must remember that the patient may have been briefed to be difficult or non-communicative.

When there is a role-player at the station, it is essential that you do not interact with the examiner who is there as an observer. If you do, this will completely break up the rapport that you have developed with the role-player. If you run out of questions and the consultation becomes silent, do not approach the examiner.

Good practice

- Introduce yourself
- Remain professional
- Stay in control of the consultation
- Ask if the patient has understood
- Ask if she has any questions
- Use diagrams/drawings if appropriate
- Practise with a friend
- A video of yourself is very useful

Clinical skills

With this type of station any skill that you perform in the wards, in the clinics or in the operating theatre can be tested, depending on the feasibility of setting up the station. These stations should be easy as it is what you do every day at work. You just need to transpose yourself mentally into the situation and do what you normally do.

Counselling skills

These stations will have a role-player and may involve breaking bad news or dealing with an anxious or angry patient. The role-players have been well briefed to act in a certain way. It is essential that you avoid medical jargon. Clearly you need to be empathetic and compassionate in these situations.

Prioritization

The ability to set priorities in clinical work – this may involve a busy labour ward, calls you may receive from the ward or the rest of the hospital, operating list priorities.

Logical thought

- The ability to design an audit, protocol, or information sheet.
- Critique of a medical journal paper, protocol or a patient information pamphlet.
- With these stations you must have an opinion as to whether the document is good or poor, and be able to defend your opinion. You must be able to give an overview of the documents, as well as addressing some details.

Clinical management of gynaecology or obstetric problems

Here you may be faced with a scenario in either the clinic or the operating theatre and you must describe to the examiner what your management would be. You may be given examination findings or results that you may need to interpret.

Communication stations

Any scenario that may occur in your working day can be tested here. At these stations knowledge is often secondary and it is how you interact with the role-player/patient that is important. If patients are angry, allow them to talk but keep control of the situation. Do not take that anger personally; they will have been told to act that way. If they are upset, let them talk, and act as though you have all the time in the world.

Structured oral examination/Viva

At these stations the examiner will ask set questions to which you need to provide the answers.

Summary

The marking of all the stations is structured and thereby objective. This means that whichever examiner you get, you should score the same mark. The examiners have practised the questions, by role-playing themselves as both the candidate and the examiner.

Global score:
- 0 = poor
- 1 = satisfactory
- 2 = average
- 3 = good
- 4 = excellent

Each station is currently marked out of 20, with four marks for a 'global' score. This takes into account your overall performance in the station and a logical approach is essential. There are no half marks. Marks will be awarded for all the tasks asked in the question.

The design of the OSCE ensures that, as far as possible, each candidate is exposed to the same examination. At the stations where there is a role-player and an examiner, do not interact with the examiner; he or she is merely an observer. To do well in the examination, all you need to do is to perform all your clinical activities as you would normally do them. It is a licensing examination and the RCOG needs to be sure you are competent.

Review Stations

Review station 1

Gynaecology history

Candidate's instructions

The patient you are about to see has been referred to your gynaecology outpatient clinic by her general practitioner. A copy of the referral letter is given below. Read the letter and obtain a relevant history from the patient. You should discuss any relevant investigations and treatment options with the patient.

The Surgery
Large Pond Road
London SE16

Dear Gynaecologist

Please would you see Joan Dunn, aged 45 years. She is a female solicitor who has a 2-year history of painful heavy periods. She bleeds for 10 days every month and is in so much pain she is bedridden throughout her period. She is fed up and wants something done.

She is overweight with a BMI of 30 kg/m^2 and on examination she has a large pelvic mass. An ultrasound scan has revealed this to be fibroids with an anterior fundal fibroid 12 × 8 × 6 cm and a submucosal fibroid 3 × 4 × 4 cm.

Thank you for your help.

Yours sincerely,

Dr W White MRCGP

MARKS WILL BE AWARDED FOR YOUR ABILITY TO TAKE A HISTORY AND TO EXPLAIN THE APPROPRIATE INVESTIGATIONS AND TREATMENT PLAN TO THE PATIENT

Role-player's instructions

You are Joan Dunn, a 45-year-old solicitor. Your attitude would be that of a friendly and calm patient who is generally interested to find out all the benefits and risks of the treatment of your problem. You may, however, turn combative if you are treated with discourtesy or belittled, or if you are generally dissatisfied with the doctor's attitude. After all, you are a busy professional woman and do not want to be treated as though you are not very bright. You are worried that you may have cancer of the womb as your sister has that problem as well.

Let the doctor know if you do not understand any medical terms. Let him lead in the discussion and do not interrupt him unless you need some clarification. You may prompt him (see below) at the end if he asks if you have any questions.

Your symptoms

- Your periods started when you were 13 years, and have been regular until recently, each period lasting about 3 days, and it comes every 28–30 days.
- However, over the last 8 months, you have noticed that you have experienced bleeding in between your periods and they are irregular. This occurs irregularly when you are expected to be dry. You have to wear pads every day and are generally worried. You do not have bleeding after sexual intercourse.
- You have seen a GP who gave you some iron tablets but these did not seem to stop your periods. No other medications were given to you.
- Your last cervical smear was done 3 years ago and that was normal.
- You have noticed that you have become more lethargic over the last 3 months, although you have not had any chest pain, shortness of breath, or palpitations.
- You have not been pregnant before as you and your husband have been rather busy with your careers and you do not intend to get pregnant.
- You have had diabetes for the last 5 years and have been very careful with your diet and the control has been good. Your yearly checks with your diabetes doctor have shown that your control has been good. You do not have any other symptoms.
- You have no drug allergy.
- There is a family history of diabetes and cancer of the womb. Your mother suffers from diabetes controlled with medication. Your sister was 39 years old when she was diagnosed with early cancer of the womb. She had an operation to remove the womb and has been well since.
- You occasionally drink alcohol and do not smoke.

Prompts

1. What condition do I have?
2. What needs to be done for me?

Mark sheet

History

- Symptoms – details of IMB
- Previous menstrual history
- Previous obstetric history
- Family history (and patient anxiety)
- Social history

0 1 2 3 4 5 6

Investigations

- FBC
- Blood glucose
- Glycosylated haemoglobin
- Cervical smear
- Pelvic ultrasound scan (ovaries and endometrial thickness)
- Pipelle biopsy of endometrium ± hysteroscopy

0 1 2 3 4 5

Further management dependent on findings

- Hysteroscopy and resection of submucosal fibroid if pipelle normal
- Hysterectomy if histology abnormal
- Low risk of malignancy (reassure patient)
- Non-hormonal treatments, tranexamic acid, mefenamic acid
- Could take cyclical hormone tablets if no specific abnormality found
- Even if nothing abnormal is found, patient encouraged to report further IMB in future
- Suggest ongoing active supervision of diabetes

0 1 2 3 4 5

Global score

0 1 2 3 4

Total: /20

Discussion

What is the station testing?

To be able to take a gynaecology history is a core skill for an MRCOG candidate. This is a skill that you practise every day and you should be very good at it. Notoriously, candidates score very badly on history-taking stations.

You are also being tested on your communication skills, so you must be sensitive to the problem but also must be very thorough in obtaining a complete history. In these stations the patients may be briefed to be difficult and may try to lead you up the wrong path. You must therefore be in control of the consultation while at the same time communicating well.

What are the pitfalls?

Most candidates are not very thorough when they take a history and, in particular, forget to enquire about family history and social history. In this day and age, one should also enquire about alcohol and recreational drug use.

At this station you have also been asked to discuss relevant investigations and treatment options with the patient. This means that you must outline the investigations, but as you are not given the results, you have to propose the treatment options depending on the results of the investigation. You must therefore be clear in your thinking as to how to get this across simply to the patient so that she can understand. It may be helpful to draw a diagram.

Preparation

As you do this every day, it is easy to practise but you need to be supervised to ensure that you are being thorough. In the exam, marks will also be awarded for being systematic rather than gleaning the information in a random fashion. The best way to practise this station is to use a real patient and ask a colleague to observe you.

Review station 2

Early pregnancy problem – management

Candidate's instructions

You are working in the early pregnancy assessment unit and the patient, Tracey Wall, you are about to see has just had an ultrasound scan. You have not met her before. The results of the scan are as follows:

Transvaginal scan Tracey Wall, aged 35, 123456

- Anteverted uterus
- Fetal pole identified in uterus
- No fetal heart activity
- Sac consistent with 5 weeks' gestation
- Both ovaries appear normal
- 25 mm corpus luteal cyst seen in right ovary

Explain the significance of this ultrasound report to the patient and the future management plan.

MARKS WILL BE AWARDED FOR YOUR ABILITY TO EXPLAIN THIS REPORT AND PLAN FURTHER MANAGEMENT

Role-player's instructions

You are Tracey Wall, a 35-year-old married barrister and you have been referred by your general practitioner for an early dating ultrasound scan having had a positive pregnancy test. You have been trying for a baby for the past 5 years and this is your first pregnancy. You have always had a regular cycle. Your last menstrual period was 7 weeks ago, but you have had a small amount of brown discharge for 10 days. Although initially delighted with the positive pregnancy test, you haven't felt pregnant for the last 4 days and you are now anxious about why the ultrasonographer would not let you see the ultrasound picture of your baby, instead asking you to see the doctor currently in the antenatal clinic.

You have had no significant medical or surgical illnesses apart from appendicitis at the age of 15 and you are taking no medication. It is now over an hour since your original appointment time and you have a work appointment very soon in your chambers. You are concerned about the ultrasound findings but also feel pressed for time, wanting a clear and confident management plan from the doctor.

You are quite a bossy woman and you are used to being in charge and telling everyone what to do. The doctor is much younger than you and you treat him like a student. You want answers and you want them now.

Mark sheet

History

- Last menstrual period, regular cycle
- First pregnancy
- Symptoms
- Focused history-taking
- Social history
- Date of pregnancy test

0 1 2 3 4

Explanation of scan findings

- Non-medical jargon
- This could be a delayed miscarriage
- This could be 5 weeks' gestation (re-checks dates)
- Cyst insignificant
- Explains that it may need evacuation
- Explains evacuation
- Management
  - offers to re-scan in a week
  - offers conservative management

0 1 2 3 4 5 6 7

Communication

- Checks she has understood
- Invites questions
- Empathy
- Deals with the way she speaks to you

0 1 2 3 4 5

Global score

0 1 2 3 4

Total: /20

Discussion

What is this station testing?

This station is testing what you would normally do with an early pregnancy problem. Miscarriage is a very common problem in early pregnancy and you should be very familiar with how to deal with this situation. You should be able to take a concise relevant history, listing important points such as last menstrual period, symptoms of pregnancy, timing of the pregnancy test and whether the pregnancy is wanted or not.

As you are dealing with a role player, you must be sensitive to her needs, and as the management path is not clear-cut, you must be able to offer alternatives and in a way be guided by her feelings. So although you are being tested on your management skills, you are also being tested on your communication skills and it is important to check that she has understood and whether she has any further questions. This situation may well be very emotionally charged and the role player may have been briefed to react to you in a certain way.

What are the pitfalls?

You must be focused to take a concise history and not spend all of your time taking a thorough history as the candidate's instructions advise you to explain the significance of the report and future management plans. However, it is difficult to do this without taking a brief history.

The corpus luteal cyst is a normal finding and you must not focus upon this as a potential problem. It is not clear-cut from the scan whether this is a viable early pregnancy of only a few weeks' gestation or whether it is a non-viable pregnancy and this must be explained to the patient. You must not be dictatorial in what you think the management should be and you must be sympathetic to what she wants.

Preparation

This is a very common problem that you are likely to encounter every week when you are on call. We are all at risk of becoming blasé about women who have miscarriages when we see them so often, but to the individual woman this can be a tragic event. It is also important to remember that one must use non-medical jargon at all times.

Review station 3

Prioritization on delivery suite

Candidate's instructions

With the following type of station you will receive the instructions at a preceding preparatory station where you will have adequate time to prepare yourself for the next station where the examiner will be. Your instructions are as follows:

- You are the registrar on call for the labour ward. You have just arrived for the handover at 08.30 h.
- Attached you will find a brief résumé of the 10 women on the delivery suite as shown on the board.
- The staff that are available today are as follows:
  - a SSHO in her 12th month of career training
  - a third-year specialist anaesthetic registrar
  - six midwives:
    - DB is in charge
    - DB, JR and BB can suture episiotomies
    - JR, DB and MM can insert an i.v. line.
- NB – the consultant on call is doing his operating list and is not keen on being disturbed unless absolutely necessary.

READ THE BOARD CAREFULLY. You have 15 minutes to decide:

- what tasks need to be done
- the priority of the cases
- who should be allocated to each task.

At the next station you will meet the examiner with whom you will discuss your decisions and your reasoning.

YOU WILL BE AWARDED MARKS FOR YOUR ABILITY TO MANAGE THE DELIVERY SUITE

Discussion

What is the station testing?

The examiner wants to assess whether you can prioritize the problems and safely manage the labour ward. You must demonstrate an organized and confident approach and be able to defend all your decisions. Do not keep on saying that you would ask the consultant's advice, as the examiner wants to know what your decisions would be. However, clearly it would be prudent to mention that you would call the consultant and check that he was happy with any operative decisions. There may be different answers to this station but as long as your decisions are sensible, you'll score well. A global score will be awarded for each room, and it is therefore important not to miss out any rooms in your conversation with the examiner. In this situation, a half mark will be rounded up.

Usually there will be one to three patients who will need urgent review, one to three who can be left for a while, and the rest will be those for whom the decision-making is important. You need to demonstrate to the examiner that you know what is important, that you have an organized mind and that you can hand responsibility over to other staff members, but you want to be informed of any problems they may encounter. Be clear and concise. Don't just repeat what is written on the board!

What are the pitfalls?

You cannot do everything! You must determine where you are needed the most and where the staff can go depending on their experience. You must delegate but ensure that the staff will communicate with you if further problems arise.

Preparation

This is an easy station to practise. Each time you walk onto a labour ward there is an OSCE station set up for you. Ideally, ask one of your seniors to spend 15 minutes with you discussing your management priorities. Practise being able to delegate duties. If you are sitting the exam at a junior level, i.e. you have never taken charge of a labour ward, ask your registrar to role-play being your junior and you do the prioritization.

DELIVERY UNIT BOARD

Room	Name	Parity	Gestation	Liquor	Epidural	Syntocinon	Comments	Midwife
1	Barnett	1+1	32	–	Yes	Yes	LSCS at 0230 (PET) EBL 800 mL baby on SCBU	DB
2	Lawson	3+0	T+9	Mec	Yes	No	8 cm at 0300 Transferred in from home	Com/MW
3	Tifou	0+0	39	Intact	No	No	Undiagnosed breech Spont. labour. 4 cm at 0730 Breech at spines	DB
4	Smith	0+0	31				Dr to see Vaginal bleeding CTG normal	BB
5	Jones	0+0	41	Mec	Yes	No	Fully at 0700	VM
6	Patel	1+0 LSCS	T+2	Clear	No	No	Trial of scar. ARM at 0300 FBS at 0600 pH 7.29 6 cm at 0600	JR
7	Finch	2+0	14	Intact	No	No	Routine admission for cervical cerelage	VM
8	Allpress	0+0	39				Delivered. Awaiting suture	MM
9	Murphy	2+0	T+6	Intact	No	No	Spont. labour 3 cm at 0650	BB
10	Grant	0+2	32	Intact	No	No	Twins. Contracting. Ceph/breech IVF pregnancy	MM

Review station 3

Examiner's instructions

The candidate has 15 minutes to explain to you the following:

A. The tasks, which need doing on the delivery suite;
B. The order in which the candidate would do them;
C. The staff he/she will allocated to each

These instructions may not be exclusive and a degree of flexibility is allowed in the marking.

Tasks required:

Room 1	Needs review post caesarean section as had severe pre-eclampsia. This review would involve pulse, blood pressure, amount of ongoing blood loss, hourly urine output and fluid status. Bloods should be repeated.
Room 2	Needs urgent review as she is a multiparous woman in her 3rd labour and should have delivered by now. She has meconium liquor and has been transferred in from home so is likely to have been in labour for a very long time.
Room 3	Needs urgent review to discuss mode of delivery and recommend epidural
Room 4	Needs assessment as to the amount of bleeding, the cause and whether or not in pre-term labour. Must exclude abruptions.
Room 5	Needs review, as should have delivered by now.
Room 6	Needs review to assess progressing adequately and review CTG and repeat FBS if any CTG abnormalities.
Room 7	Needs non-urgent review and consent to be signed after fetal viability has been checked and dating of the pregnancy has been re-checked
Room 8	Needs suturing.
Room 9	Needs review later in the morning when the other cases have been sorted out.
Room 10	Needs urgent review as may be in premature labour. If she is in premature labour, she will need steroids with tolcolysis.

The priorities for review are: Room 2 is the first priority, followed by Room 3 and Room 10 and then Room 4. It would be appropriate for the Registrar to see Room 2 and Room 10 and the SHO to see Room 4 and Room 3. The midwife could suture Room 8 and Room 9 could be assessed by the midwife later in the morning. After the urgent cases have been sorted out, then the medical staff should review Room 6 and Room 5.

Mark sheet

Room 1	0	1	2	3	4
Room 2	0	1	2	3	4
Room 3	0	1	2	3	4
Room 4	0	1	2	3	4
Room 5	0	1	2	3	4
Room 6	0	1	2	3	4
Room 7	0	1	2	3	4
Room 8	0	1	2	3	4
Room 9	0	1	2	3	4
Room 10	0	1	2	3	4

Total **/40 → divide by 2**

Final mark **/20**

Review station 4 ✓

Surgical skills – placenta praevia

Candidate's instructions

You have admitted a 32-year-old primigravida for an elective Caesarean section. She has major placenta praevia and the presentation is breech. She is currently 38 weeks' pregnant.

The examiner will ask you a series of five questions regarding aspects of this woman's care following her admission, i.e. counselling, preparation, techniques, postoperative care and follow-up. You will need to highlight issues related to Caesarean section in general as well as those related to this specific case.

THIS IS A STRUCTURED VIVA. YOU WILL BE TESTED ON YOUR ABILITY TO APPRECIATE PREOPERATIVE, INTRAOPERATIVE AND POSTOPERATIVE MANAGEMENT OF A MAJOR OBSTETRIC PROCEDURE

Mark sheet

The candidate has been given the task of arranging an elective Caesarean section for major placenta praevia. Please ask the following questions:

'Preoperatively what will you discuss with the patient?'

- Site of placenta (anterior, posterior)
- Risks, benefits, consent
- Warn about need for i.v. line, catheter, possible drain, possible blood transfusion
- Type of anaesthesia

0 1 2 3

'What other personnel will you liaise with?'

- Anaesthetist, paediatrician, haematologist
- ODA/midwife
- Partner (warn of seriousness of operation)

0 1 2 3

'Preoperatively what will your orders be?'

- Nil by mouth for > 6 hours
- Intravenous fluids, antibiotics, ranitidine, shaving, catheter, TED/Flowtron stockings
- Blood available in theatre

0 1 2 3

'Take me through your operative procedure and outline any concerns'

- Consultant involvement
- Incision – abdominal, uterine (classical vs. lower uterine), oxytocin, morbid adhesion of placenta, closure
- Quick entry through placenta and clamp cord immediately
- Be prepared for excessive blood loss

0 1 2 3 4

'Postoperatively what would you do?'

- Ensure adequate i.v. fluids
- Check haemoglobin
- Hourly urine output initially
- TED stockings
- Thromboprophylaxis
- Early mobilization
- Discuss future pregnancies
- Contraception

0 1 2 3

Global score

0 1 2 3 4

Total: /20

Discussion

What is the station testing?

This woman is about to have a potentially life-threatening operation. The examiner wants to know what you would normally do before a Caesarean section as well as the extra precautions that you would take in this case. You must be thorough and go through your normal checklist, appreciating that with this type of case a lot of extra preparation is required so that the operation can be as safe as possible.

What are the pitfalls?

You must be aware of the seriousness of the case. No matter how experienced one is, this type of case can bleed excessively and be very frightening for all concerned. It is easy to miss out obvious precautions and concentrate on the more dramatic features, thus failing to carry out routine preparation.

Preparation

Design difficult scenarios and ask your colleague to play the examiner. When a difficult surgical case occurs in your clinical practice, go back to the beginning and see if you could have been better prepared so that the case was easier.

Review station 5

Communication skills – ectopic pregnancy

Candidate's instructions

The patient, Flora Burton, you are about to see has returned to the emergency gynaecology unit for follow-up after an operation for an ectopic pregnancy 14 days ago. She had a salpingostomy and the ultrasound today has shown a live ectopic on the left side.

Please explain the results of the ultrasound scan to her, suggest management and answer her questions.

MARKS WILL BE AWARDED FOR TAKING A RELEVANT HISTORY, DISCUSSING A MANAGEMENT PLAN AND ADDRESSING HER CONCERNS

Role-player's instructions

You are Flora Burton, a 35-year-old woman who had your last menstrual period 9 weeks ago. This pregnancy has not been straightforward: from 6 weeks onwards you had some vaginal bleeding and at 7 weeks you presented to the early pregnancy unit and were told that you had an ectopic pregnancy. You had a laparoscopy and the tube was opened up and the ectopic was removed. You were told to return the following week to check that the pregnancy levels had gone down but you didn't do this and you have continued to have some bleeding. Now you have some pain on the left side. When you presented today to the early pregnancy unit, they performed another scan and did another blood test. You do not know the results of the scan or the blood test but you are just about to see a doctor who will explain the ultrasound scan to you and suggest further management.

You will be told that the ectopic still remains in the left tube when you thought the operation had removed it. You are clearly very cross about this as your previous obstetric history has not been straightforward. You want to know why the pregnancy was not removed 2 weeks ago and you are now terrified that the hospital is going to make another mistake (with your first pregnancy, from which you now have a 3-year-old child, you were originally told it was ectopic, you had a laparoscopy and it turned out to be an intrauterine pregnancy). You are therefore adamant that you do not want them to put anything into the womb when they do a further operation until they are absolutely sure that it is a persistent ectopic pregnancy.

You are obviously extremely upset about what has occurred and you are very cross that the pregnancy wasn't removed in the first place. You would like to see the person who operated on you first immediately so that you can express your displeasure.

As you are now looking at a further laparoscopy, you want conservative treatment for that tube as you do not want to rule out all possibility of a future pregnancy – your second pregnancy was a right ectopic pregnancy which was removed by laparotomy 18 months ago.

You and your husband very much wanted this pregnancy and you are not quite sure how you are going to tell him all this bad news. You suspect that he is also going to be cross as he cares so much about you.

You are otherwise fit and well and you take no medications and don't smoke or drink alcohol. You have no family history of any significant diseases and you are not allergic to anything.

Mark sheet

History

- Previous ectopic pregnancy – laparotomy
- Previous normal pregnancy originally thought to be ectopic
- Current pregnancy thought to be ectopic and had laparoscopic salpingostomy 2 weeks ago

0 1 2 3 4 5

Management plan

- Explains ultrasound findings and its implications
- Needs a laparoscopy – encourages salpingectomy, however, accepts her wish for conservative surgery
- Accepts her wish for non-manipulation of the uterus

0 1 2 3 4 5

Communication

- Explains that persistent ectopics can occur with laparoscopic conservative surgery for tubal ectopics
- Does not blame previous surgeon for supposed negligence
- Diffuses situation as much as can
- Discusses IVF for future pregnancies

0 1 2 3 4 5 6

Global score

0 1 2 3 4

Total: /20

Discussion

What is this station testing?

This is a difficult situation where a previous operation has not been correctly performed. This station tests your ability to diffuse a situation where a woman is clearly very angry while at the same time not 'bad-mouthing' one of your colleagues. With regard to her anger, it is better to allow her to get angry at you and get it off her chest, and it is best for you to be a passive listener.

However, you do have to manage the case and you need to be quite clear in telling her what needs to be done, but you also need to accept her wish for a more conservative approach with regard to instrumenting the uterus and conservative surgery on the tubes. You also need to be quite clear that if she opts for conservative surgery again, not only is there a very small chance of the trophoblastic tissue persisting, but also, in the future, she has a further chance of an ectopic. If she was going for IVF then it is in her interests to have this tube removed.

What are the pitfalls?

It is very easy to say that the previous operation was not done correctly but you need to avoid saying this. You must take a focused history, as her past pregnancy history is very important here. There are therefore three aspects to this station and one of the pitfalls is not to cover them all. You need to take a focused history, explain what needs to be done now and discuss the prognosis for future pregnancies and how you can help her.

Preparation

These stations are difficult to prepare for because they do involve patients who are quite angry because something has gone wrong. The best way to practise this station is to ask a colleague to role-play the angry patient and try to deflate the situation.

Review station 6

Premenstrual syndrome

Candidate's instructions

The patient you are about to see has been referred to your outpatient clinic by her general practitioner. A copy of the referral letter is given below.

Read the letter and obtain a relevant history from the patient. You should discuss any relevant investigations and treatment that you feel may be indicated.

Dear Gynaecologist

Re: Mrs Jodie Revell – DOB 23.06.70

I would be pleased if you would see this patient who has coerced me into referring her for a gynaecological opinion. She says that she has severe premenstrual symptoms. She does not seem to have responded to anything that I have prescribed her.

Many thanks.

Yours sincerely

Dr A. N. Other

YOU WILL BE MARKED ON YOUR ABILITY TO TAKE A RELEVANT GYNAECOLOGY HISTORY AND DISCUSS INVESTIGATIONS AND TREATMENT OPTIONS

Role-player's instructions

You are Jodie Revell, currently 34 years old, and you are completely fed up. You have terrible premenstrual symptoms and you have been to your GP many times for this but he just tries to fob you off. Your main symptoms are mood swings, irritability, pelvic pain and sometimes violent behaviour. Your relationship is almost in tatters because your partner is fed up with your behaviour. You are perfectly lovely for 3 weeks out of 4, but for 7 days before your period you turn into a completely different person.

You have had an episode of depression in the past but you don't believe that there is anything psychiatrically wrong with you. You have been violent in the past and certainly have hit your partner on numerous occasions. You have tried the odd vitamin for premenstrual syndrome (PMS) but nobody has ever really explained it to you and you are just very fed up. You work as an assistant to a dental surgeon and you do find it extremely stressful as the practice is a very busy private practice and, as well as working very hard, you have to be sweet and nice to everybody all of the time otherwise your boss gets upset because his private practice, and therefore his income, is also dependent on your personality.

You had an unwanted pregnancy 6 years ago and you had a termination. You are currently using the mini-pill for contraception but you appear to have regular periods. You had chlamydia about 3 years ago and you have been with your current partner for 5 years. It always worried you that he had deviated when you found out that you had chlamydia.

You have no past medical or surgical history of note. Medications you take are Neurofen Extra premenstrually for the pelvic pain. You smoke 20 cigarettes a day and drink about 20 units of alcohol per week. You enjoy the odd joint of marijuana and have about three per week.

Family history – your mother suffered from severe depression and has been on antidepressants for some years.

Examiner's instructions

At this station, candidates will have 14 minutes to obtain a history relevant to the patient's complaint. They should ask about clinical examination and then investigations that they think may be relevant, explaining them to the patient along the way. They should also discuss possible treatments.

Mark sheet

History

- History taking to elicit the actual symptoms
- Important to establish that the symptoms are definitely premenstrual and disappear by the end of the period
- Elicits the patient's concerns about how the symptoms are affecting her home and professional life

0 1 2 3 4 5

Investigations

- appreciates that there are no relevant investigations
- explains this to patient

0 1 2

Management

- Establishing the diagnosis by a symptom/visual analogue diary
- Hierarchy of treatments
  - counselling/education/reassurance/stress management and relaxation techniques
  - pyridoxine/essential fatty acids
  - selective serotonin reuptake inhibitors (SSRIs) – ensure that used specifically for PMS and not depression in this case
  - OCP/progesterone/danazol
  - oestradiol patches (or implants) + cyclical progesterone
  - gonadotrophin-releasing hormone (GnRH) analogues ± back therapy
  - total abdominal hysterectomy (TAH) and bilateral salpingo-ophorectomy (BSO) followed by oestrogen hormone replacement therapy (HRT)

0 1 2 3 4 5 6 7

Communication

- Discusses management in a non-confrontational and empathic way
- Emphasizes attempts at stopping ovulation

0 1 2

Global score

0 1 2 3 4

Total: /20

Discussion

What is the station testing?

As with the station concerning antenatal history-taking, this station is testing your communication skills and ability to take a comprehensive gynaecology history of a difficult problem. In the referral letter, the GP has stated that he was not happy to refer her on to a specialist, so there are clearly problems in the interaction between the patient and her GP. This indicates that this will not be an easy consultation and you will need to be particularly good at communicating and being empathetic.

Clearly you must concentrate on her symptoms of PMS, but in a station like this it is very important that you enquire as to the effect on family, friends and work.

What are the pitfalls?

One can infer from the letter that this patient is quite desperate to receive help for this problem. She will therefore have very high expectations from the consultation and may be very emotional and have a low threshold for becoming aggressive and/or tearful. As with the antenatal history, you need to be thorough in asking about all the different histories and to be sure to include social and drug history, which includes recreational drugs. You should also do a systems functional enquiry. Many candidates are not organized in the way they extract information.

If the patient does become aggressive then you must defuse the situation, and at the end of the consultation you must ensure that the plan of management is clear and ask her if she has any further questions, emphasizing the next point of contact.

Preparation

As with the antenatal history, you need to practise taking gynaecology histories and this can be easily done in pairs. Be systematic in how you take the history, as this will determine your global score in the examination. Where clinical examination is not mentioned, you should assume it is normal, otherwise it would have been included in the question.

Review station 7

Breaking bad news – anencephaly

Candidate's instructions

You are the registrar in the Department of Obstetrics & Gynaecology. Mrs Ruth Barker, aged 28 years and pregnant for the first time, is having a scan at 16 weeks' gestation following a raised serum alpha-fetoprotein (AFP) result. The radiographer has detected that the fetus has anencephaly and has called you in, as the patient is booked under your consultant's care. You agree with her observations and have been asked to counsel Mrs Barker about these findings.

You are about to meet Mrs Barker and there is no doubt about the diagnosis. You have 14 minutes to counsel her about the situation.

MARKS WILL BE AWARDED FOR:

- Explaining the diagnosis
- Discussing options open to the patient
- Dealing with the patient's concerns

Role-player's instructions

You are Mrs Ruth Barker, a 28-year-old woman who has been referred for a scan because of an abnormal blood test (raised serum AFP – the spina bifida blood test) and so you have had an inkling that something is not quite right.

It seems that all is not well, as the radiographer has called in a doctor and the doctor has suggested you discuss things in a separate consultation room. The doctor will tell you that your baby has anencephaly (the head and brain have not formed properly) and that this is incompatible with life. You will question the doctor about the options open to you, including further tests, a second opinion and the outlook for the baby if you decide to continue the pregancy.

You are a devout Roman Catholic and need to see your priest and partner before making any decision. You ask about the possibility of organ transplantation if you carry the baby to term.

You are naturally upset and concerned about the possibility of future pregnancies and how you are going to cope with it mentally, whatever you do.

This is your first pregnancy and you have been trying to become pregnant for a few years. Otherwise you are fit and well with no family history of any significant diseases.

Mark sheet

Explaining the diagnosis

- Explains the results, avoiding jargon
- Explains that the rise in serum AFP was an indication for a scan
- Diagnosis in little doubt but would she like a second opinion
- Allows patient to express concerns, shock and confusion

0 1 2 3 4

Discussing the options

- Offers options of termination or continuing pregnancy
- Timing of termination unlimited by the Abortion Act, 1991
- Discusses the mechanics of the termination:
  - intracardiac potassium chloride (possible)
  - mefipristone tablets orally and then a series of five cervagem pessaries after 36 hours
  - a further course may be needed if the first course does not work.
  - extra-amniotic if this procedure does not work
  - risk of requiring an evacuation of the uterus afterwards for retained placenta
  - pain relief, as the pains are similar to labour pains

0 1 2 3 4

- If continuing pregnancy, discusses problems:
  - routine antenatal care would need to be undertaken
  - risk of postmaturity as fetal pituitary stimulates onset of labour and this is likely to be absent
  - difficult to get into labour as nothing pressing on the cervix
  - need for operative delivery may be necessary if shoulders are difficult to deliver or if there is delay

0 1 2 3 4

Patient concerns

- Gives them the option to come back after time to think it over
- Postmortem examination may be useful
- Arranges for any appropriate counselling both before and after delivery
- Consequences for a future pregnancy, recurrence rate 1 in 30
- Use of folic acid beneficial in a future pregnancy
- Organ donation – would need to seek advice, but practically it is not likely to be an option

0 1 2 3 4

Global score

0 1 2 3 4

Total /20

Discussion

What does this question test?

This question is concerned with the candidate's ability to counsel a patient and break bad news. The scenario is such that there is no doubt about the diagnosis. You need to divide your time equally between the three parts of the question. This situation is really the application of knowledge plus experience. It is appreciating that anencephalic pregnancies may progress and that there are inherent risks of postmaturity and difficulty in delivering the shoulders. It is important to provide support and not judgment; forewarned is forearmed and patients will not automatically opt for termination. A decision does not need to be arrived at by the end of the consultation. However, options need to be provided, including coming back with a partner or supporter.

The examiner will check the candidate's number and there will be no other interaction – the examiner has a purely marking role.

The role-player will have been given the scenario. She has been given key points to test candidates' ability to apply their knowledge to the situation. The question about organ donation is one that has been asked of the author, but advice would need to be sought as organs can only be removed when the donor has died, making this a difficult area ethically. If candidates are unaware of any policies then they should explain that advice would need to be sought. This approach will be reflected in the global score as to how they have dealt with the situation.

What are the pitfalls?

The major pitfall in all counselling questions is that the candidate fails to read the question properly and consequently does not answer it. When in doubt candidates revert to history-taking with which they feel comfortable. No history is required here; it is not relevant. There is no doubt about the diagnosis, but there is a tendency for candidates to give erroneous information to the role-player. It is also important to know the local protocol and apply it to the scenario. It is necessary to empathize with the role-player, but important information needs to be communicated and candidates should always be mindful of what exactly they are being asked to do, as the marking scheme will reflect those tasks. A good candidate will be aware of the distress a diagnosis like this may cause – termination may not necessarily occur with the first course of cervagem as the patient is a primigravida, and continuation of the pregnancy is not without its risks. A good candidate is likely to draw a diagram to explain the diagnosis to illustrate to the patient exactly what is the problem.

Advice and preparation

There are three parts to this question, the main one dealing with whether to terminate or continue this pregnancy. It is important, as with all the OSCEs, to utilize your time appropriately. In the examination you are given a pad to take round with you, and in this situation drawing a diagram may be a very useful way of conveying some of the information, as it can be difficult to get the role-player to take it on board from a solely verbal explanation. It is important to remember that this news can be devastating for the patient, and one should avoid 'okay' and 'all right' and keep checking that the role-player understands the significance of what you are saying.

This station is very much the 'appliance of science', i.e. the application of your obstetric knowledge to deal with a bad news scenario. Imagine this is a clinic situation and do what you would do there. Prior to the OSCE part of the MRCOG, it would be useful to sit in with a senior colleague when they are breaking bad news if you have no experience of doing so. It is important to allow the role-player to have time to speak as she may furnish you with valuable information. Do not be afraid of silences, providing they do not go on for too long. The role player will have been briefed to ask questions if you have come to a halt.

What variations are possible for this question?

Breaking bad news in the obstetric scenario can be very variable, from fetal abnormality (fatal or non-fatal), intrauterine fetal death or stillbirth. In all these scenarios there will be no doubt about the diagnosis and marks will be awarded for dealing with the situation and not history-taking.

Review station 8

Infertility – case notes

Candidate's instructions

This is a preparatory station and you have 15 minutes to review the notes and results of the patient you will see in the next station.

The patient and her partner were referred to your outpatient clinic by her general practitioner. They were originally seen in the clinic 3 months ago and some baseline investigations were undertaken. The original notes have been lost. A copy of the original referral letter has been found plus a copy of the original clinic letter. Copies of the results have also been placed in the notes.

YOU WILL BE AWARDED MARKS FOR:

- Discussing appropriate supplementary history
- Discussing results of investigations
- Discussing appropriate treatment options

The Surgery,
Blackhorse Rd,
London E44

Dear Doctor

Can you please see Susan Pesh who has a history of infertility over the past 3 years?

Susan is 27 years old with a history of mild endometriosis, which was diagnosed laparoscopically 2 years ago. The endometriotic spots were found on the uterosacral ligaments only and these were diathermied. The rest of the pelvis appeared normal. Susan has been on a course of Provera for 6 months and is now asymptomatic.

Regards

Dr Twort

Dear Dr Twort

Re: Susan PESH (7.7.73)
26, Victoria Gardens, E44

Thank you for referring this patient to my gynaecological outpatients' clinic with a history of primary infertility. She commenced her periods at the age of 13 years and appears to have a regular 28-day cycle with bleeding for 5 days. The rest of her gynaecological history is unremarkable except for a previous history of endometriosis that appears to have been successfully treated with ? at the time of laparoscopy and Provera. She is now asymptomatic. Her coital frequency appears to be satisfactory. Her smears are up to date and normal. The rest of her medical history is unremarkable and she is not taking any medication.

General physical examination was unremarkable with a BP of 110/70 and a normal BMI. Pelvic examination was normal.

I have organized some routine investigations and plan to see her again in 3 months' time when the results should be available. I will keep you informed of her progress.

With best wishes

Yours sincerely

Mr A Sherman

Day 21 progesterone (Susan PESH 7.7.73)
60 IU/L (follicular 0–15 IU/L)
(luteal > 25 IU/L)

Hysterosalpingogram (Susan PESH 7.7.73)

- The uterus is normal anteverted and mobile. Both uterine tubes fill and the isthmus and ampullary portions appear normal
- There is free spill of contrast into the peritoneal cavity bilaterally with little retention of dye

Pelvic USS (Susan PESH 7.7.73)

- Normal anteverted uterus, with normal looking ovaries
- No pelvic pathology seen and no evidence of PCO
- Small amount of fluid in the POD

HVS result (Susan PECK 7.4.62.)
Normal commensals plus *Candida* spp.

Endocervical swab (Susan PESH 7.7.73)
Negative for *Chlamydia*

Semen analysis (Brian PESH, partner of Susan PESH 7.7.73)

Collection	Masturbation
Days abstinence	1 day
Time since production	90 minutes
Volume	2.8 mL
Viscosity	Normal
Motility	30%
Sperm concentration	0.6 million/mL
Abnormal form	50%
Non-sperm cell conc'n	0.3 million/mL
Total motile sperm	0.5 million
Tray agglutination test	No antisperm antibody detected

Repeat semen analysis (Brian PESH, partner of Susan PESH 7.7.73 – 2 months later)

Collection	Masturbation
Days abstinence	5 days
Time since production	30 minutes
Volume	4 mL
Viscosity	Normal
Motility	35%
Sperm concentration	0.9 million/mL
Abnormal form	55%
Non sperm cell conc'n	0.1 million/mL
Total motile sperm	2.4 million

Role-player's instructions

You are a 27-year-old woman called Susan Pesh who works as a sales assistant. You commenced your periods at the age of 13 years and now have a regular 28-day cycle with bleeding for 5 days. You are unsure about when you ovulate but only volunteer this information if asked. You have been with Richard, your husband, for 5 years and have regular intercourse, three times a week.

Apart from a laparoscopy as an investigation for pain on intercourse you have had no other surgical procedures. You were treated for mild endometriosis, although you are a little unsure about the nature of it. The rest of your history is unremarkable, you are a non-smoker and you are not taking any medication. Your last smear was prior to your referral and the result was normal. You have used the oral contraceptive pill in the past but at the age of 21 for 9 months only.

Your partner is likewise fit and well and works as a panel beater. He is a non-smoker and drinks a glass of wine with meals. He does, however, like to smoke marijuana at least once a week. He has not had any previous testicular problems and has not fathered a child.

You are getting anxious and depressed because all your family are expecting you to get pregnant as easily as your two sisters and all your school friends are on at least their second baby by now.

The results would suggest that there is a male factor and so the candidate should explain the various technologies available for you. You feel your partner may get very distressed at the thought that it is probably his problem and not yours.

Mark sheet

Appropriate supplementary history

- May ask about LMP
- May ask if partner has had any testicular problems, tumours, infections, operations
- Asks about smoking, alcohol and any recreational drugs of patient and partner
- May ask about type of underwear and bathing habits of partner
- Any previous children
- May check about coital frequency
- May ask about *Candida* and if she has had treatment or is still symptomatic (wrong name)

0 1 2 3 4 5

Discusses investigations and relevance

- Ovulating normal midluteal progesterone
- Fallopian tubes patent on the HSG
- Infection status negative for *Chlamydia* but positive for *Candida* (wrong name)
- Semen results shows main problem is with a low sperm count
- Further count may be useful but diagnosis is unlikely to be different
- Notices wrongly labelled result

0 1 2 3 4 5

Discusses appropriate treatment options

- Never say that the patient can never get pregnant, but may have difficulties
- Advises to stop marijuana, usual advice about underwear, baths and multivitamins
- Advises that IUI may not be very successful
- Donor insemination may not be the first line of treatment
- Suggests reproductive technologies IVF/ICSI
- NICE guidelines suggest IVF should be available on the NHS
- Asks patient how far does she want to proceed and adoption may be an option

0 1 2 3 4 5 6

Global score

0 1 2 3 4

Total /20

Discussion

What does this question test?

This question has a preparatory station in order to allow the candidate to read the case notes. However, it could be placed at the station to go through with the patient present which would simulate what can happen in reality. The question is looking at whether the candidate can interpret the clinical findings and results. This is the kind of scenario in which one may find oneself in a clinic, with very basic information and copies of letters. It is unlikely that there will be a role-play couple. You may have to counsel either the woman or her partner in a similar situation. It could be the man who you are seeing to discuss his sperm count and this may lead to a very confrontational consultation. The actors will have been primed to ask specific questions in order to lead you along the mark sheet of the examiners.

There are three aspects to what is required and it is important to think of relevant questions related to the low sperm count. With all infertility questions, there will usually be an obvious diagnosis. It is always important to find out how far along the road of assisted treatments a couple is prepared to go.

The examiner will be in place to award marks and nothing else.

What are the pitfalls?

The major pitfall is in answering the question, being critical of the notes and allowing yourself time to deal with all three tasks. This is clearly a case of infertility due to a male factor. It is important that the candidate has a clear idea of the normal values of the common tests that are undertaken in the gynaecological outpatient clinic. In most cases, the normal ranges will be given, but even so the candidate should know the normal range of any test requested. This is particularly true in obstetrics when the normal range may change due to the pregnancy. As in real life, it is important to check that the results belong to the patient in front of you. There may be results that have been deliberately labelled incorrectly and these need to be identified. This is especially true if you are breaking bad news.

Advice

There are three parts to this question. In the preparatory station it is worth making notes of specific parts of the history that have not been addressed or documented to date. These would revolve around any possible reasons for a low sperm count, e.g. drugs, history of previous children, and other social issues. The second part of the question is to interpret the results to the patient and that can only be done if normal values are known. The third part of the question is to discuss the low sperm count and the specific options that may be useful for this case. You would need to have a clear idea about the options and how to get access to them.

What variations are possible for this question?

Alternatives to this question would be endocrinology cases where a number of results are given to the candidate and those results have to be interpreted by the gynaecologist. As the examination may occur over 2–3 days, comparable stations will need to be found for each day, e.g. different causes for infertility, secondary amenorrhoea, etc.

Review station 9

Audit

Candidate's instructions

A copy of an algorithm that is used in the early pregnancy assessment unit is supplied. This protocol was instituted in an attempt to reduce the number of unnecessary ultrasound scans performed.

Discuss with the examiner how you would design an audit to ascertain how well this protocol is being adhered to, and what steps you would take if the audit revealed that overall compliance is poor. You are not being asked to comment or criticize the protocol as such.

YOU WILL BE AWARDED MARKS FOR:

- Discussing the factors you would take into consideration
- Designing an audit to address the question
- Discussing how you would use the results

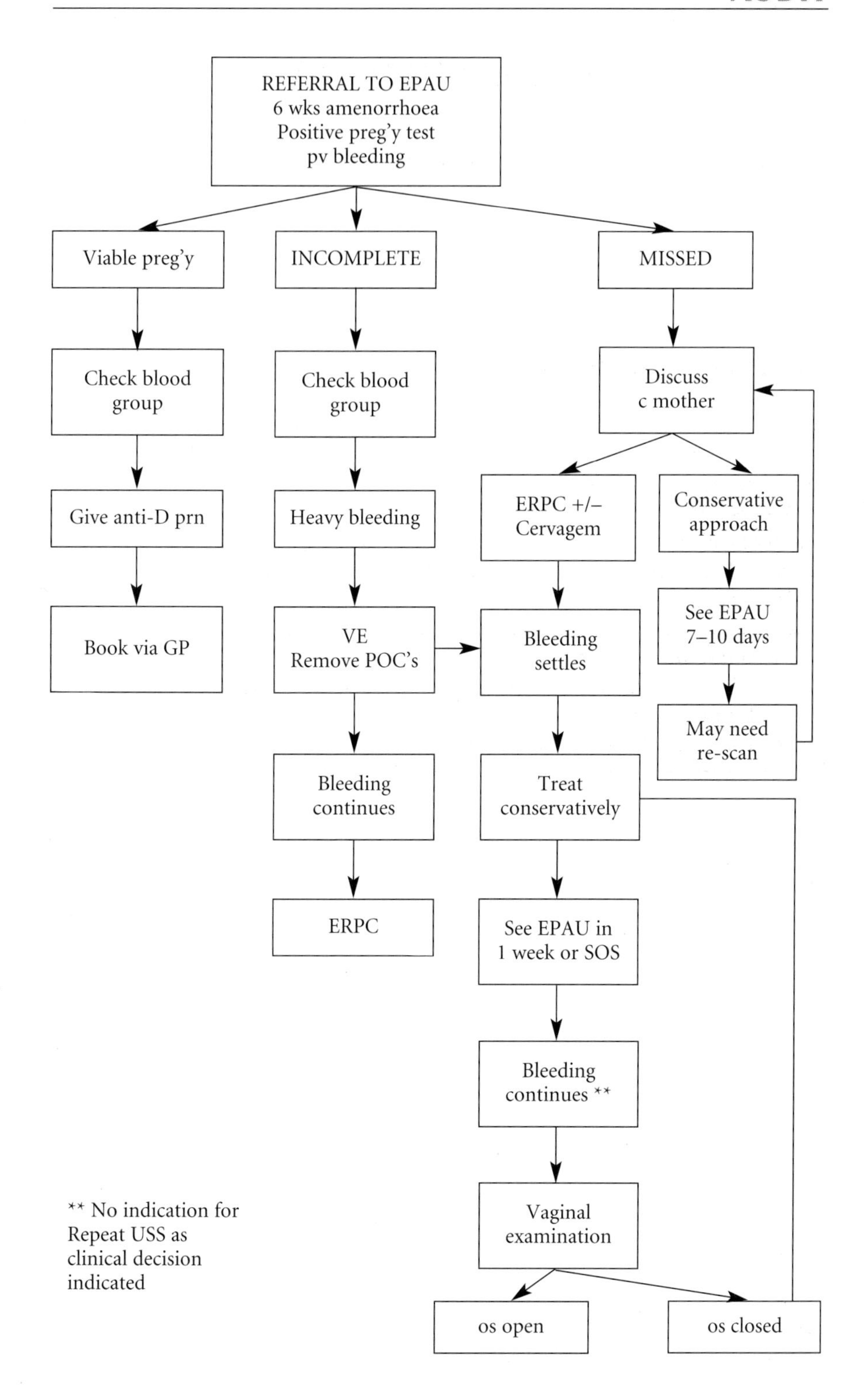
REFERRAL TO EPAU
6 wks amenorrhoea
Positive preg'y test
pv bleeding
Viable preg'y
INCOMPLETE
MISSED
Check blood group
Check blood group
Discuss c mother
Give anti-D prn
Heavy bleeding
ERPC +/– Cervagem
Conservative approach
Book via GP
VE Remove POC's
Bleeding settles
See EPAU 7–10 days
May need re-scan
Bleeding continues
Treat conservatively
ERPC
See EPAU in 1 week or SOS
Bleeding continues **
Vaginal examination
os open
os closed
** No indication for Repeat USS as clinical decision indicated

Examiner's instructions/mark sheet

Candidates need to cover the following areas of discussion and can be prompted by a specific question if they do not mention them spontaneously.

Factors to be considered

- Which patients should have been managed?
- Evidence-based medicine
- RCOG/national guidelines
- Consumer interaction/expectation

0 1 2 3 4

Design the audit

- Determine sample size
- Establish a data sheet/proforma to identify patients' course
- Define outcome
- Identify missing data and eliminate bias
- Identify key failures in following the algorithm

0 1 2 3 4 5 6

Use of results

- Feed results back to staff at regular audit meeting; may need to talk to GPs or hold meetings for relevant stakeholders
- Anticipate reactions
- Hard on the issue, soft on the individual; avoid a blame culture
- Consider necessary organizational changes to improve or allow compliance
- Resource implications may be an issue
- How to achieve consistent implementation
- Time taken for changes to be implemented
- Decide when audit should be repeated
- Completing the audit cycle
- Change in protocol may not make further audit data comparable

0 1 2 3 4 5 6

Global score

0 1 2 3 4

Total **/20**

Discussion

What does this question test?

This question is designed to test the candidate's understanding of audit. The algorithm or protocol is relatively immaterial. It is not the protocol that is being criticized but the adherence to the protocol that is being tested. There may be a preparatory station prior to meeting the examiner. The examiner will expect the candidate to go through the steps of an audit cycle. If the examiner has to prompt the candidate then the marking will be reflected accordingly.

What are the pitfalls?

The major pitfall in this type of question is not understanding the audit process and instead spending the time criticizing the protocol. All UK trainees are expected to undertake some form of audit during their posts and this is the place to learn how to do it. You need to be aware of proforma or data sheets that need to be produced and whether the audit should be done on a numbers basis or over a specified time. That will reflect the frequency of the condition. For early pregnancy problems, it may be useful to do the next 200 cases; if the subject was water birth then it may be worthwhile using a fixed time period. Most audits should be done prospectively as there is a risk of losing cases if done retrospectively, which may alter the ultimate outcome.

Advice

The following is a way of undertaking an audit. It is useful for candidates to have undertaken an audit within their own organization.

- Agree audit scope and objectives
- Audit methodology/design
- Review current practice
- Agree preferred practice
- Design proforma/audit tool
- Collect data
- Analyse data
- Conclusions/recommendations
- Action plan
- Re-evaluation

Review station 10

Obstetric history

Candidate's instructions

The patient you are about to see has been referred to your antenatal clinic by her general practitioner. A copy of the referral letter is given below. Read the letter and obtain a relevant history from the patient. You should discuss any relevant investigations that you feel may be indicated.

The general physical examination of the patient should be taken to be unremarkable.

Dear Doctor

Would you please book Andrea Rollings for antenatal care? She is 11 weeks' pregnant. I have enclosed some of the investigation results.

Yours sincerely

Dr Beattie

(Andrea ROLLINGS 2.6.78)

- FBC – normal
- Blood group – O, Rh-positive
- VDRL – negative
- Rubella – non-immune
- MSU – no growth
- USS – single live intrauterine pregnancy consistent with 11 weeks' gestation. No other abnormalities detected

YOU WILL BE MARKED ON:

- Obtaining an obstetric history
- Establishing risk factors for this pregnancy
- Discussing relevant and appropriate investigations

Role-player's instructions

You are Andrea Rollings, a 27-year-old woman who works in the sex industry. You are single and live alone. Your periods are regular every 28 days with a 5-day bleed. You had been using the combined oral contraceptive pill (OCP) and this pregnancy was due to a pill failure. You are unsure of the date of your last menstrual period and don't see it as relevant when you know that the recent scan makes you 11 weeks' pregnant. This is your first pregnancy and you have a certain amount of ambivalence towards it. You are also off-hand with anyone you see as an authority figure. You don't make the interview easy, as you view the doctor in this way. Your personal/medical information is as follows:

- Medical and surgical history – nil of note
- Last cervical smear 5 years ago
- Smokes 20/day
- Alcohol – three whiskies/day
- Recreational drugs – marijuana and cocaine but nothing intravenously
- Medication and allergies – nil

Examiner's instructions

At this station, candidates will have 14 minutes to obtain a history relevant to the patient's complaint. Candidates should also discuss with the patient any relevant investigations they feel are appropriate.

Investigations that need to be considered are as follows:

- Hepatitis B and C screen
- HIV test
- Cervical smear
- HVS and *Chlamydia* swabs

Mark sheet

Obstetric history

- Basic obstetric history, including LMP, cycle length, EDD
- Previous medical and surgical history and any family history of note
- Is it planned and does she want to continue with the pregnancy?
- Deals with social factors, looking at alcohol, cigarette and recreational drug consumption
- How is the pregnancy progressing to date?

0 1 2 3 4 5 6

Risk factors

- Brings out the fact that she may be at risk of HIV and substance abuse
- How is she supporting her habits?
- Asks about occupation
- Emphasizes the importance of attending for routine antenatal check-ups

0 1 2 3 4

Relevant investigations

- Routine investigations already done, including FBC, group, rubella, syphilis
- Talks about Down's screening
- HIV screening
- Cervical cytology (opportunistic)
- *Chlamydia*
- Hepatitis B and C

0 1 2 3 4 5 6

Global score

0 1 2 3 4

Total /20

Discussion

What does this question test?

This question tests the ability of the candidate to take a basic obstetric history and, in so doing, establish the risks for this patient and her pregnancy. Once the correct questions have been asked, any relevant investigations and appropriate management should ensue. It is looking at a patient who has a high risk of sexually transmitted disease, risk of an abnormal smear and also the possibility of drug abuse and the problems that may ensue in a pregnancy. The examination is taken to be normal and so there should be no interaction with the examiner, whose role is to mark according to the prescribed mark sheet. The role-player has been given a scenario and will answer questions when asked. She will have been briefed as to how much help to give candidates and in some cases will have specific questions to ask candidates in order to help them with the questions. If the question does not have a bearing on the scenario, the role-player will answer that all is normal.

What are the pitfalls?

The major pitfall in an obstetric history-taking station is that, in the UK, a midwife takes most full obstetric histories so the candidate is not in the routine of taking a history. Key points are not asked, e.g. whether this was a planned pregnancy, occupation, menstrual history and smear history. A lot of antenatal care involves routine screening and it is important to appreciate this fact when it comes to taking a history. It is important to elicit risk factors, including tobacco and alcohol consumption. It is important to ask about 'recreational drugs' and it is best asked in those terms. As with any pregnancy, a plan of action needs to be formulated and a decision arrived at as to whether the pregnancy is high or low risk. Another major pitfall that arises in many of the role-playing stations is the use of medical jargon and especially abbreviations. The role-players are non-medical, in order to simulate a real clinic setting, and they may not understand medical terms. They will pick you up on this, making you feel rather silly for using such words.

Advice

This patient may seem to be a nightmare patient but it is important to go back to the instructions and what is required. Get into the habit of taking routine obstetric histories and formulating plans for the pregnancy in the 14 minutes allocated. It is also useful to go through booking notes in antenatal clinic to assess risk factors.

Most history-taking questions are relatively straightforward, although in an OSCE situation there may be some kind of twist in the story. The role-player may have been primed to ask appropriate questions to steer you on track.

Be aware of the routine screening blood tests that are performed in the UK.

Circuit A

Circuit A, Station 1

Breaking bad news – cancer

Candidate's instructions

You are the registrar in the gynaecological outpatient clinic and you are about to see Ms Kylie Spears, a 40-year-old single woman who underwent a hysteroscopy and curettage 2 weeks ago and is here to obtain the results. She has had a history of heavy, irregular vaginal bleeding for the past 3 months and was treated by her GP with a course of oral contraceptive pills with no relief. She was subsequently referred to this hospital for further investigation. Below is the histology report.

Please counsel Ms Spears. THIS IS A COUNSELLING STATION.

Four Mills District Hospital, Leicestershire

Department of Pathology

Patient name: Kylie Spears
ID no.: T7785254
Age: 40
Date: 28 December 2004
Specimen: endometrial curettings

Histology report
Moderately differentiated adenocarcinoma of the endometrium

Verified by:

....
Dr Nisha Khan
MRC Path.

YOU WILL BE MARKED ACCORDING TO YOUR ABILITY TO EXTRACT THE RELEVANT HISTORY AND EXPLAIN THE DIAGNOSIS AND TREATMENT

Role-player's instructions

- You are Ms Kylie Spears, a 40-year-old primary school teacher.
- You are single, not sexually active and will be married to your fiancé, Richard, in 6 months.
- You love children and plan to have three.
- You currently live with your parents and three brothers and you are close to your family.
- Your menarche (first period) was at age 10. Your periods are irregular with each cycle lasting 1–6 months. Your periods last 4–5 days and are not heavy. You have mild, tolerable dysmenorrhoea. You have always thought this pattern of periods was normal.
- You have never used contraception and have never had a cervical smear.
- You have not taken any regular medication except in the last 3 months.
- You have not noticed any weight changes but have always been chubby. You have not noticed any increased hair growth.
- You do not smoke, and drink socially occasionally.
- Four months ago, your periods suddenly became frequent, occurring every few days and heavy with clots.
- There was no abdominal pain.
- You saw your GP, who prescribed a course of the combined oral contraceptive pill for the past 3 months.
- The medication reduced the flow of the periods but there was still daily vaginal spotting.
- You were then referred to this hospital for a hysteroscopy and D&C.
- You are well after the D&C. There are no abdominal pains or vaginal discharge but you continue to have daily vaginal spotting.
- You are worried about the result of the operation.
- You are extremely upset about learning of the cancer, especially when you are to be married and plan to have children.
- You are suspicious that your GP had treated your symptoms conservatively for 3 months and that that time had made a difference to the stage of the disease.

Prompt questions

- What is the result of the operation, doctor?
- Is it cancer? Is it curable?
- Is there no way for me to have children in the future?
- Why has this happened to me?
- What are the risks of the surgery?
- What are the risks and side-effects of radiotherapy?
- Why didn't my GP refer me earlier – I may not have got cancer?

Mark sheet

Relevant history

- Menstrual history – previous irregular, long cycles, never took medication except the OCP in the last 12 months
- Risk factors – no diabetes mellitus, non-smoker, non-drinker, nulliparous
- No family history of any cancers
- Fertility desires – to be married in 6 months. Wants to have children
- Social support – financially stable. Good family support. Good relationship with parents and siblings
- No previous medical/surgical history

0 1 2 3 4

Explanation of histological report

- Malignancy of lining of womb
- Extent of disease unknown. Will need MRI prior to surgery
- Need for total hysterectomy and bilateral salpingo-oophorectomy, possible lymph node dissection
- Surgery procedure – GA, midline or phannenstiel incision and risks of surgery, i.e. anaesthetic risks, venous thromboembolism, bladder, bowel injury, bleeding, infection

0 1 2 3 4

Discusses consequences of treatment

- No further fertility, menopause and consequent risk of osteoporosis, climacteric symptoms
- Risk of HRT
- Prognosis depends on staging. Varies from 95 per cent in stage 1 to 10 per cent in stage 4
- May need postoperative radiotherapy depending on histology
- Will need co-management with gynae-oncologist and treatment in a gynaecological cancer centre or unit dependent on MDT review

0 1 2 3 4 5

Counselling

- Addresses patient's concern about GP's initial conservative management
- Offers counselling to cope with news

0 1 2 3

Global score

0 1 2 3 4

Total mark: /20

Circuit A, Station 2

Preoperative ward round

Candidate's instructions

You are the registrar responsible for the following morning's operating list. Your consultant will be in the hospital but has an important meeting and would prefer not to be disturbed. You now have to do the preoperative ward round. There are three patients on the list:

- Mrs Andrews – a 42-year-old for a total abdominal hysterectomy
- Mrs Devine – a 35-year-old for a diagnostic laparoscopy
- Mrs Norman – a 35-year-old for a resection of a submucosal fibroid.

You are about to meet the examiner. He will ask you some questions about what you would normally do with each patient preoperatively.

Examiner's instructions

Please ask the candidate the following:

- Mrs Andrews is 42 years old with a 20-week fibroid uterus for a total abdominal hysterectomy.
  - What relevant history do you want to know?
    - what symptoms she is having?
    - is she still premenopausal?
    - previous surgery?
    - has subtotal been discussed?
  - What results of investigations would you like to know?
    - USS
    - Hb
    - pregnancy test
    - cervical smear
  - What would you discuss with her?
    - does she know what operation she is having?
    - confirm ovarian conservation has been discussed
    - discuss incision – vertical
  - What would you warn her of?
    - haemorrhage
    - bowel/bladder trauma
    - catheter postop
    - i.v. line
    - drain
  - Anything else you would do?
    - examine her abdomen
    - ask if she had any questions

0 1 2 3 4 5 6

- Mrs Devine is a 33-year-old woman who is having a laparoscopy for right-sided pelvic pain (? endometriosis).
  - What relevant history do you want to know
    - nature of pain
    - exact site of pain
    - past O&G history
    - past surgery
  - What results of investigations would you like to know?
    - USS
    - Hb
    - pregnancy test
    - cervical smear
  - What would you discuss with her?
    - does she know what operation she is having?
    - if endometriosis is found diathermy would be useful

- What would you warn her of?
  - bowel/bladder trauma
  - where incisions will be
- Anything else you would do?
  - examine her abdomen
  - ask if she had any questions
  - go through consent form with her

0 1 2 3 4 5

- Mrs Norman is a 35-year-old woman who has a 3-cm-diameter submucosal fibroid that has been causing her regular heavy periods.
  - Any relevant history you would like to know?
    - any previous O&G history
    - any previous surgery
  - What results of investigations would you like to know?
    - Hb
    - USS
    - pregnancy test
    - cervical smear
  - What would you check she has had preoperatively?
    - GnRH agonists
  - What would you warn her of?
    - uterine perforation which would then require a laparoscopy
  - Anything else you would do?
    - examine her abdomen
    - ask if she had any questions
    - go through consent form with her

0 1 2 3 4 5

Global scale

0 1 2 3 4

Total score **/20**

Circuit A, Station 3

Obstetric history and management

The patient, Shirley Wright, you are about to see has just been admitted to your maternity unit. The midwife is concerned about her and no other doctor is available to see her at present. You have 14 minutes to obtain a history from the patient and outline the plan of management.

THIS STATION TESTS YOUR ABILITY TO TAKE AN OBSTETRIC HISTORY AND YOUR COMMUNICATION SKILLS WITH REGARD TO MANAGEMENT

Role-player's instructions

- You are 39 years old and this is your second pregnancy and you have reached 26 weeks' gestation:
  LMP = 29 weeks earlier
  EDD = 11 weeks later
- This pregnancy is the result of in vitro fertilization and intracytoplasmic sperm injection (third attempt) after 5 years of infertility due to severe problems with the quality of your partner's sperm.
- Your first pregnancy was at the age of 17 and you had a termination.
- You booked at the maternity hospital at 12 weeks' gestation.
- Triple test at 15 weeks, risk of Down's syndrome 1 in 175.
- Serum AFP within normal range.
- Chorionic villous sampling at 11 weeks uneventful. Result – normal male karyotype.
- Ultrasound at 18 weeks normal.
- The day before admission you felt generally unwell, (feverish, tired). Several hours prior to admission you experienced a gush of fluid vaginally and there has been persistent vaginal dampness since.
- Now aware of lower abdominal cramps.
- Personal – married, secretary.
- Family – mother has IDDM.
- Sister with spina bifida, sister had DVT while on OCP.
- Social – smoke 10 cigarettes/day.
- < 5 units of alcohol per week.
- Drugs – folic acid.
- PMH – congenital dislocation of the hip as a baby, and have had recurring hip problems since.

Role-player's attitude

You are very worried about your situation and fear that you are going to lose your baby. You continually seek reassurance from the doctor.

Mark sheet

History

- Personal details – TOP
- Family history:
  - IDDM
  - NTD
  - DVT
- Social history – smoker
- Previous menstrual history
  - CDH
  - infertility

0 1 2 3 4

Presenting complaint

- Gestation
- Premature rupture of membranes
- Contractions?
- Sequence/timing

Current pregnancy

- IVF + ICSI
- LMP/EDD
- AFP/triple test
- CVS
- Ultrasound scan

0 1 2 3 4

Management

- Admit
- Steroids
- Regular scan
- Monitor WBC, CRP
- CTG
- Expectant management
- Antibiotics

0 1 2 3 4

Communication

- Empathetic
- Concise but clear information
- Arranges neonatal paediatrician to visit
- Allows patient to express anxieties

0 1 2 3 4

Global score

0 1 2 3 4

Total score /20

Circuit A, Station 4

Management problem – gynaecology

Candidate's instructions

A 45-year-old nulliparous female solicitor, Ms Marianne Brighton, has been referred to you by the GP complaining of painful heavy periods. She bleeds for 10 days every month and has so much pain that she is bedridden throughout her period. She has regular cervical smears, all of which have been normal.

Four years ago she had a lumpectomy for breast cancer and is now on tamoxifen. She smokes 20 cigarettes a day and is otherwise well. She is fed up and wants something done.

You have examined her and found:

- BMI = 30 kg/m^2
- Soft, obese, distended abdomen
- 18-week-sized irregular abdomino-pelvic mass, confirmed to be fibroids on ultrasound scan – anterior fundal fibroid (12 × 8 × 6 cm); submucosal fibroid (3 × 4 × 4 cm).

You are about to see the patient. Ask her relevant questions and then outline the options, discussing any risks involved.

MARKS WILL BE AWARDED FOR YOUR ABILITY TO TAKE A RELEVANT HISTORY AND DESCRIBE MANAGEMENT OPTIONS

Role-player's instructions

- You are Ms Marianne Brighton, a 45-year-old solicitor.
- For the last 3 years you have had very heavy menstrual periods, bleeding for 10 days every month and the pain throughout the periods is unbearable. You even go to bed during your periods as the pain is so bad.
- Periods are regular.
- You have been told that your womb is enlarged and sometimes you feel that there is pressure on your bladder as you have to pass urine frequently.
- You have never tried to get pregnant as you still have not met the right man. You have had partners in the past but none at the moment. You accept that you may not get pregnant and will consider a hysterectomy.
- You are pretty well but 4 years ago had breast cancer and had a lumpectomy and you have been on tamofixen ever since.
- You have had regular Pap smears, which were normal.
- You smoke 20 cigarettes a day.
- Allergic to amoxil – you get a rash.
- Family history of ovarian cancer – mother and maternal aunt.

Mark sheet

Enquires about the relevant past history

- Past obstetric and gynaecological history – nulliparous
- Other treatments that have been tried?
- Stable relationship?
- Prospects for children? Is family complete?
- Pressure symptoms?

0 1 2 3 4

Which surgical procedure (need endometrial biopsy first)?

- Hysteroscopy – resection of submucosal fibroid may be an option
- Myomectomy
- Subtotal hysterectomy ± Bilateral salpingo oopherectomy (BSO)
- Total abdominal hysterectomy ± BSO
- Other options:
  – arterial embolization
  – do nothing

0 1 2 3 4

Risk of procedures

Immediate
- Anaesthetic
- Bladder/bowel injury
- Haemorrhage
- Risk of unwanted hysterectomy (for hysteroscopy and myomectomy)

Intermediate
- DVT/PE
- Bladder problems
- Infection

Long term
- DVT/PE
- Bladder problems
- Psychosexual – loss of womanhood

0 1 2 3 4

Advantages and disadvantages of procedures

- Hysteroscopy – less invasive but may need further procedure as pressure symptoms won't be improved
- Myomectomy – will preserve fertility but must understand chance of hysterectomy and massive bleeding
- Subtotal hysterectomy – (+ total abdominal) both may have premature menopause; subtotal is the easier operation, there are fewer bladder problems postoperatively and ?better sexual function; however, cervix remains – potential site of cancer, ? may still bleed
- Other options – still in research arena

0 1 2 3 4

Global score

0 1 2 3 4

Total: /20

Circuit A, Station 5

Prenatal counselling

Candidate's instructions

You are the registrar in the antenatal clinic. Please see Ms Anna Reid, a 35-year-old Caucasian woman who has been married for the past year and is planning her first pregnancy. She is keen to find out more about genetic testing for cystic fibrosis. You are asked to take a relevant history from this patient and address her concerns.

YOU WILL BE MARKED ON YOUR COMMUNICATION SKILLS AND YOUR ABILITY TO EXPLAIN TO HER ABOUT THE DISEASE OF CYSTIC FIBROSIS AND THE RISKS OF HER BABY BEING AFFECTED WITH CYSTIC FIBROSIS

Role-player's instructions

Profile

- You are Ms Anna Reid. You are 35 years old, married for the past year and are now keen to start a family. You have never been pregnant before.
- You are Roman Catholic by religion.
- A few months ago, your mother revealed to you that she had a brother who was affected with cystic fibrosis before she was born and passed away at age 6 years, before you were born.
- Your periods are regular, normal flow, no dysmenorrhoea. Your last cervical smear was 12 months ago and was normal. You have not used any form of contraception.
- You have no medical/surgical history of note.
- Your husband, Alan, is aged 40 and is a Caucasian. He is Protestant by religion.
- As far as you know, his family has no history of cystic fibrosis.

Concerns about the disease which need to be addressed

- You are worried about the possibility of your child being affected with cystic fibrosis.
- You would like to know more about the disease.
- You would like to know whether you are a carrier.
- You would like to know if the disease can be detected in the baby and how it can be tested.
- You would like to know how accurate is the testing.

Mark sheet

Relevant history

- Age, parity and religion – 35 years old, para 0, Roman Catholic
- Family history – mother has revealed to her that she had a brother who was affected with cystic fibrosis before she was born and passed away at age 6
- No medical/surgical history of note
- Husband's age and race – aged 40 and is a Caucasian
- History of cystic fibrosis in husband's family – none of note

0 1 2 3 4

Explanation of the disease

- Inherited disease, inherited in an autosomal recessive manner
- Affects lungs, digestion and reproduction
- Basic problem is in the production of mucus and saliva, which leads to recurrent chest infections, indigestion and malnutrition. Intelligence is normal
- Chronic condition requiring prolonged care and multiple hospital visits
- Life expectancy – 20s to 30s

0 1 2 3 4

Chance of baby being affected

- A child is affected if he or she inherits one affected gene from each parent and has two abnormal genes
- With the history of her brother being affected, Ms Reid is either normal with no affected genes or a carrier with one affected gene
- If she and her husband are both carriers, then the risk of the baby being affected is 25 per cent. The risk of the baby being a carrier is 50 per cent and the baby has a 25 per cent chance of being normal

0 1 2 3

Genetic testing

- In a Caucasian population, the chance of a person being affected is 1 in 25.
- Parental testing can be done to determine if a person is a carrier
- Genetic testing identifies up to 90 per cent of all cystic fibrosis gene spontaneous mutations and may miss 10 per cent of mutations

- Testing if the baby is affected allows the parents to know if the pregnancy is affected and, if so, allows termination of the pregnancy if they are not prepared to care for such a child
- Fetal testing can be done by testing the baby's cells via one of two methods: amniocentesis or chorionic villous sampling

0 1 2 3 4 5

Global score

0 1 2 3 4

Total: /20

Circuit A, Station 6

Obstetric emergency – uterine inversion

Candidate's instructions

You are the registrar in charge of the labour ward. You are urgently called by the midwife. She has just discovered that a patient who had a vaginal delivery has collapsed.

YOU WILL BE MARKED ON YOUR ABILITY TO ANSWER THE EXAMINER'S QUESTIONS REGARDING THE EMERGENCY OUTLINED AND TO EXPLAIN HOW YOU WOULD SYSTEMATICALLY MANAGE IT

Mark sheet

You arrive in the room and the midwife is there with the uterus inverted and placenta attached. The examiner's questions are as follows:

'What are your immediate management actions?'

- This is an obstetric emergency and the candidate will go and see the patient immediately
- Activate emergency code to mobilize SHO, anaesthetist, charge midwife
- Establish and maintain airway of patient, begin chest compression if asystole. An intravenous line should be started and blood for FBC, urea/electrolytes, liver function test, coagulation profile, uric acid level, hypocount, group and save should be taken

0 1 2 3 4

'What is the subsequent management of this patient?'

- Prompt gentle replacement of the uterine inversion manually – last out/first in method
- Use of uterine relaxant, e.g. i.v. terbutaline 0.25 mg, or general anaesthesia in the operating theatre
- Hydrostatic method (O'Sullivan's method) – the inverted uterus is held within the vagina and warm saline infused (about 2 L is infused rapidly into the vagina)
- If still unsuccessful, may need emergency laparotomy and replacement of uterus by traction on round ligaments
- As a last resort, a Caesarean hysterectomy may be necessary
- Once stable, correction of anaemia or coagulopathy with blood and fresh frozen plasma, if necessary
- Use of oxytocin drip should be started to maintain uterine contractility
- Observation in high-dependency unit for hourly BP, HR and urine output measurements
- Antibiotic cover should be started
- TED stockings

0 1 2 3 4 5 6 7 8

'Other management steps?'

- Inform consultant
- Inform patient's partner or next of kin and warn them of preventive steps at next delivery, i.e. controlled cord traction with fundal guarding in the third stage of labour
- Record the events systematically and chronologically in the case notes
- Record the events in an 'incident report' form

0 1 2 3 4

Global score

0 1 2 3 4

Total: /20

Circuit A, Station 7

Operating list – prioritization

Candidate's instructions

You are asked to go through a consultant's gynaecology waiting list and advise the waiting list manager on:

- appropriate procedure(s) (operation and others)
- venue of proposed treatment (outpatients department, day unit, in-patient)
- special needs (if any)
- priority of assignment – routine (within 6 months), soon (within 12 weeks), urgent (within 4 weeks).

Please describe your action and offer an explanation wherever appropriate. You will have 15 minutes to review this list and will discuss it at the next station with the examiner.

YOU WILL BE AWARDED MARKS FOR YOUR ABILITY TO MANAGE AND PRIORITIZE THE CASES

Waiting list for operations (candidate's information)

Name	Age	Details	Operation and logical action	Venue	Special needs	Priority
JA	28	Deep dyspareunia, menorrhagia, ovarian cyst (8 cm) (scan suggests benign cyst)				
AB	42	Large pelvic mass. Likely ovarian cyst CA125 = 45 IU/mL				
JF	18	Recent abnormal smear. Cervical biopsy CIN3. Requests treatment under GA				
PH	30	P3+1. Recent TOP. History of subacute-bacterial endocarditis and DVT. Wishes laparoscopic sterilization				
PR	18	Primary amenorrhoea/cyclical pain. Ultrasound – distended vagina				
KR	32	P5+0. Missing IUCD. Caring for invalid child (IUCD in abdominal cavity)				
QT	44	Fibroid uterus. Menorrhagia. Haemoglobin 8.1, Jehovah's Witness				
TN	82	Recent angina. Procidentia/lives alone/incontinent (failed pessary)				
TL	28	Laparoscopy for pain, previous laparotomy (twice)				
JB	22	Secondary subfertility – 3 years. Previous ectopic				

Examiner's information

Waiting list for operations

Name	Age	Details	Operation and logical action	Venue	Special needs	Priority
JA	28	Deep dyspareunia, menorrhagia ovarian cyst (8 cm) (scan suggests benign cyst)	Hysteroscopy and laparoscopic ovarian cystectomy	Day unit		Soon
AB	42	Large pelvic mass. Likely ovarian cyst CA125 = 45 IU/mL	Laparotomy. Consultant must be present	In-patient		Urgent
JF	18	Recent abnormal smear. Cervical biopsy CIN3. Requests treatment under GA	LLETZ	Day unit		Soon
PH	30	P3+1. Recent TOP. History of subacute-bacterial endocarditis and DVT. Wishes laparoscopic sterilization	Laparoscopic sterilization, antibiotic cover, anticoagulant	Day unit		Soon
PR	18	Primary amenorrhoea/cyclical pain. Ultrasound – distended vagina	Incise hymen	Day unit		Urgent
KR	32	P5+0. Missing IUCD. Caring for invalid child (IUCD in abdominal cavity)	Laparoscopy? Proceed laparotomy (consultant)	In-patient, but home same day if possible	Good notice	Soon
QT	44	Fibroid uterus. Menorrhagia. Haemoglobin 8.1, Jehovah's Witness	LHRH analogues, iron tablets, embolization, subtotal hysterectomy	In-patient		Soon
TN	82	Recent angina (failed pessary). Procidentia/lives alone/incontinent	Vaginal hysterectomy, needs preoperative assessment	In-patient	Arrange postoperative care	Soon
TL	28	Laparoscopy for pain, previous laparotomy (twice)	Laparoscopy (consultant present)	In-patient	Warn re. risk of bowel damage	Routine
JB	22	Secondary subfertility – 3 years. Previous ectopic	Laparoscopy dye, endometrial biopsy	Day unit		Routine

Mark sheet

Discuss each case briefly with regard to:

1. Logical action (operation and others)
2. Venue of proposed treatment
3. Special needs
4. Priority assignment

Global score

JA	0	1	2	3	4
AB	0	1	2	3	4
JF	0	1	2	3	4
PH	0	1	2	3	4
PR	0	1	2	3	4
KR	0	1	2	3	4
QT	0	1	2	3	4
TN	0	1	2	3	4
TL	0	1	2	3	4
JB	0	1	2	3	4

Total: **/40 → divide by 2**

Final mark **/20**

Extra notes

The answers are not clear-cut so one needs to confirm that there is a common-sense approach, and this should be reflected in the global score for each case.

- AB – it should be clear that a consultant must be present for this operation.
- KR – this operation might be successfully done laparoscopically but if this proves impossible, a laparotomy may be necessary. The operative arrangements should reflect this, so it may be best to admit her as an in-patient on the understanding that, if a laparotomy proves unnecessary, she might go home on the same day. The special needs arrangement for the care of her invalid child would have to reflect the 'worst' scenario. Does she need the operation at all?
- QT – the operation could include either TAH or subtotal TAH (not myomectomy). The candidate should discuss the preoperative treatment of the anaemia and the prerequisite of a normal blood count prior to surgery. Although oral iron may be sufficient, the discussion should also include hormonal ovarian suppression if this fails. The special operation consent form is best done prior to admission.
- TN – the use of anaesthetic preoperative assessment should be discussed.
- TL – this patient is best admitted as an in-patient because of the possibility of bowel damage during laparoscopy. She should be warned of this risk.
- JB – is this appropriate? Will need *Chlamydia* screening and prophylaxis.
- JA – check CA125.
- PH – mirena inserted under antibiotic cover may be a safer option.

Circuit A, Station 8

Bereavement

Candidate's instructions

Mrs Tina Shoe was a 26-year-old primigravida who presented to the labour ward with a 24-hour history of decreased fetal movements at 39 weeks' gestation. At that time her general observations were normal. Unfortunately the fetal heart could not be heard and an intrauterine fetal death was confirmed by ultrasound scan.

The pregnancy had been classed as 'low risk' and antenatal care provided by the community midwife and the GP. She had considered a home delivery. She was a bit of a worrier and had experienced some abdominal pain and had a CTG 24 hours prior to admission. At the time this was reported as normal, but on review it was less than optimal. She had been sent home.

Following the diagnosis of fetal demise, labour was induced and after 12 hours Mrs Shoe delivered a 2.3 kg macerated stillborn male infant with the cord wrapped tightly around the neck. The patient's postnatal course was a little stormy, as her blood pressure was quite labile, rising to 140/100 with 2+ proteinuria. This settled after 36–48 hours.

At this station you will meet Mrs Shoe's husband, who has come to see you 6 weeks after the event. His wife is physically well but has gone to stay with her mother in Bournemouth. The husband is very angry and is demanding an explanation for the death of his son.

Postmortem has shown an anatomically normal male infant weighing 2.3 kg. All fetal and maternal investigations were normal.

MARKS WILL BE AWARDED FOR YOUR ABILITY TO DEAL WITH A DIFFICULT SITUATION AND TO COUNSEL AN ANGRY BEREAVED PERSON

Role-player's instructions

You are Mr Shoe and work as a window cleaner. You are at your wits end. Your wife has had a stillborn baby and she blames herself for it. She is a worrier and continued to smoke throughout the pregnancy but only 10 cigarettes/day. She has had to go to her mother's house, as she cannot cope at home when you are out at work. This event has put a real strain on the marriage and you feel she may never try for a baby again in case the same thing happens. Certainly sex is out of the question at the moment so you have to relieve yourself and you are getting fed up with it.

You cannot understand how this happened as the pregnancy had been considered low risk and you had even thought about a home delivery. You want to know if the midwife and GP did not provide the appropriate care. The baby seemed very small and you can't understand why that wasn't picked up – after all, she seemed to be down at the antenatal clinic for hours at a time. Why hadn't she had more scans?

Questions/remarks

- 'Why did this happen when she had some monitoring the day before and the doctor at that time said everything was all right?'
- 'Who is to blame and what are you going to do about it?'
- 'I'm going to complain and go to the papers. This shouldn't happen in this day and age. I am going to sue this hospital.'
- 'I want to see the boss man.'

Mark sheet

Communication skills

- Appropriate introduction
- Sympathetic approach – not responding aggressively
- Expression of sympathy
- Allowing husband to talk – not interrupting
- Asking about his wife and how they are coping as a couple
- Maintaining eye contact
- Trying to defuse anger

0 1 2 3 4 5 6

Dealing with the case

- Recognizing IUGR
- Fetal demise may have been due to IUGR which may have been PET-induced
- Cord around fetus may be causal or incidental
- Explanation of postmortem findings, avoiding medical jargon
- Advice for future pregnancy, including aspirin, folic acid, serial scans

0 1 2 3 4 5

Advice/comments

- Not incriminating colleagues
- Not becoming agitated at mention of suing
- Explain access to complaints procedure
- Offer to meet again with his wife and the carers
- Offer to discuss management in a further pregnancy

0 1 2 3 4 5

Global score

0 1 2 3 4

Total: /20

Circuit A, Station 9

Emergency contraception

Candidate's instructions

The patient you are about to see has attended the gynaecological ward for emergency contraception. She is Ruth Hale and is 31 years old. You are the registrar on call and the staff on the ward would like you to see her as they are short-staffed and, due to bed shortages, the ward is full of elderly patients. They are very busy and unable to deal with this patient unless she waits a considerable time.

MARKS WILL BE AWARDED FOR:

- Taking an appropriate history
- Counselling her appropriately
- Discussing appropriate examinations

Role-player's instructions

You are Ruth Hale, a 31-year-old librarian. You live at home with your aged parents but were coerced into going out on a hen party last night. You got a bit drunk and became quite disinhibited. Your friends set you up with the male stripper who had been the entertainment at the party, which was held in one of your colleague's houses. One thing led to another and you had unprotected intercourse with him. This is unusual behaviour for you as you have only had one sexual partner in the past, and that was soon after you finished university.

Your last period was 2 weeks ago, your cycle is usually about 28–30 days and you usually bleed for 5 days. You have never had any pregnancies or gynaecological problems in the past. You do, however, suffer intermittently from migraine. You have no known allergies and are not taking any medication.

It is now about 12 hours since you had intercourse and you are still a little hung over and also disinhibited, so may be a bit crude and graphic about what happened.

You do not feel you could cope with the embarrassment of being pregnant at this stage in your life, although you would love to become pregnant at some stage.

Questions

- 'What methods are there?'
- 'What is the failure rate?'
- 'What happens if it fails, would it affect the baby?'
- 'You won't have to examine me will you?'
- 'This is confidential isn't it?'

Examiner's instructions

History

- LMP and check it was normal
- Patient's cycle
- Calculate date of ovulation
- Hasn't had sex for many years
- Days in the cycle of unprotected sex
- Number of hours since episode of unprotected sex
- Current method of contraception
- Any potential contraindications

0 1 2 3 4 5 6

Counselling

- Methods available, mode of action and risks
- Levonelle better efficacy than PC4, 0.75 mg × 2, 12 hours apart, or IUD time limit 5 days
- Failure rate and implications
- Attitude to possible pregnancy if method fails
- Importance of follow-up
- Make final decision about PCC
- Warn about action if vomiting occurs (if within 2 hours with levonelle then take second dose and get a repeat prescription)
- Discuss contraception in current cycle
- Long-term contraception needs
- Keep accurate records, time and date
- Discuss STD screening

0 1 2 3 4 5 6 7

Vaginal examination

- May reveal concealed pregnancy
- May reveal possible infection
- Do microbiological swabs
- IUD suitability

0 1 2 3

Global score

0 1 2 3 4

Total: /20

Circuit A, Station 10 ✓

Intermenstrual bleeding

Candidate's instructions

The patient you are about to see has been referred to your outpatients clinic by her general practitioner. A copy of the referral letter is given below.

Read the letter and obtain a relevant history from the patient. You should discuss with the patient any relevant investigations and management options that you feel may be indicated.

The Surgery
Lauriston Rd,
Hackney
London E9

Dear Doctor

Re: Hetty Buckingham 23-07-70

Would you please see this patient who seems to have been getting some intermenstrual bleeding over the last 12 months. She has a BMI of 23 and pelvic examination was normal and, in particular, the cervix looked normal.

Yours sincerely

Dr A.P. Rilfool MRCGP

MARKS WILL BE AWARDED FOR:

- Taking an appropriate history
- Discussing appropriate investigations
- Discussing appropriate management options

Role-player's instructions

- You are Hetty Buckingham, a 34-year-old accountant in a stable relationship. You have a 4-year-old son who was a normal delivery and he weighed 3.2 kg.
- You have been on the OCP (microgynon) for many years and it has always suited you. You were recently diagnosed as epileptic and started on some medication for this condition. You are vague about the epilepsy and only mention it if asked. You are currently taking carbamazepine 200 mg daily. You have noticed recently that you have become a bit forgetful and occasionally forget to take the odd OCP.
- You and your partner are not keen on a further pregnancy.
- You have noticed over that past 3–6 months that you have had some intermenstrual bleeding but no postcoital bleeding. Your periods are otherwise regular every 28 days, bleeding for 4–5 days. You are otherwise well and asymptomatic. No previous history of note except for some degree of irritable bowel syndrome.
- You also want to explore with the doctor some other form of contraception. You are unsure of your last smear test – both the result and when it was performed.

Mark sheet

History-taking

- Length IMB occurs in cycle
- Any postcoital bleeding
- Ellicits history of epilepsy
- Carbamazepine
- Wants to consider other contraception
- Pregnancy history and not wanting further children

0 1 2 3 4 5 6

Investigations

- Do another pelvic examination to do a cervical smear
- Arrange a USS

0 1 2 3

Management

- Discusses fact that OCP may not be high enough dose with carbamazepine which interferes with absorption

0 1 2

- Discuss either:
  - increasing the dose of OCP
  - IUCD
  - mirena
  - depoprovera
  - sterilization

0 1 2 3 4 5

Global score

0 1 2 3 4

Total: /20

Circuit B

Circuit B, Station 1

Labour ward prioritization

Candidate's instructions

You are the registrar on call for the delivery unit. You have arrived for the handover at 08.30 h. Attached you will find a brief résumé of the 10 women on the delivery suite as shown on the board.

The staff who are available today are as follows:

- a second-year O&G SHO
- a second-year anaesthetic registrar
- the on-call consultant, who has been asked to deal with a problem in main theatres
- six midwives:
  - SW is in charge
  - SW, CK and MC can suture episiotomies
  - DB, SW and PL can insert i.v. lines.

Read the board carefully. You will have 15 minutes preparation for this station and will discuss it with the examiner at the next station.

MARKS WILL BE AWARDED FOR:
• Detailing tasks to be done • Prioritizing the cases • Allocating staff to each task

RM	NAME	PARA	GEST	LIQUOR	EPID	SYNT	COMMENTS	MW
1	SMITH	0+1	32	C	N	N	SROM 4 days ago. Dexamethasone given Contracting 1 in 3 since 0300hrs	SW
2	JONES	2	41	–	–	–	Delivered 0600 hrs. N.V.D. Bleeding	SW
3	HOWARD	1+0	39	C	N	N	Breech in spontaneous labour 6 cm at 0600 hrs	VM
4	GREEN	0+1	40	C	Y	Y	Fully dilated at 0600 hrs CTG non re-assuring	CK
5	SPENCER	2+0	38	–	–	–	Delivered, awaiting suturing	CK
6	BAKER	2	34	I	–	–	Abdo pain & vomiting. CTG normal Doctor to see	DB
7	NGOSA	3	37	I	N	N	Due for elective CS at 39/52 Admitted contracting & scar tenderness	DB
8	COLGATE	0+0	36	I	N	N	Twins contracting regularly 4 cm dilated Ceph/Breech	MC
9	McMILLAN	1	39	MEC	Y	N	ARM 0300 hrs – CTG suspicious pH at 07–30 was pH 7.23 – 6cm	PL
10	DAVIS	2	41	C	N	N	Spontaneous labour 6cm at 0500 hrs Domino	Comm MW

CIRCUIT B

Examiner's instructions

Candidates have 15 minutes to explain to you the following:

- the tasks that need doing on the delivery suite
- the order in which they would do them
- the staff they will allocate to each.

These instructions may not be exclusive.

Tasks required

- Room 1 – TPR, needs assessment; paediatricians need to be informed, can SCBU cope with the baby
- Room 2 – needs assessment, TPR, i.v. line, bloods, fluids, catheter. Assess amount of blood loss, placenta complete? May need EUA, clot expulsion, the four Ts: tissue, tone, trauma and thrombin
- Room 3 – needs reassessment, for vaginal delivery, CTG status, may need epidural
- Room 4 – needs assessment, ?delivery or FBS. Has she been pushing, or undelivered because epidural v. effective?
- Room 5 – midwife to suture
- Room 6 – assess, needs more history, MSU/dipstick, examination, previous obs history, possible non-obstetric cause for pain, e.g. appendix
- Room 7 – needs assessment, bloods and consent, will need CS. Is the CTG normal?
- Room 8 – needs epidural, monitoring both twins, bloods, routine observations
- Room 9 – needs assessment, repeat FBS
- Room 10 – no action.

Priority of tasks

There may not be total agreement with these suggestions. As long as there is consistency and safety, one can score according to how confident one is of the candidate's priority setting:

- Urgent review: rooms 2, 3 and 4
- Semi-urgent review: rooms 7 and 9
- Routine review: rooms 1, 5, 6, 8 and 10.

Personnel

Room 1 – SHO
Room 2 – reg
Room 3 – reg
Room 4 – reg
Room 5 – midwife
Room 6 – SHO
Room 7 – SHO/reg
Room 8 – SHO
Room 9 – SHO/reg
Room 10 – midwife

Mark sheet

Room 1	0	1	2	3	4
Room 2	0	1	2	3	4
Room 3	0	1	2	3	4
Room 4	0	1	2	3	4
Room 5	0	1	2	3	4
Room 6	0	1	2	3	4
Room 7	0	1	2	3	4
Room 8	0	1	2	3	4
Room 9	0	1	2	3	4
Room 10	0	1	2	3	4

Mark **/40 → divide by 2**

Final mark **/20**

Circuit B, Station 2 ✓

Abdominal pain – premature labour

Candidate's instructions

The patient you are about to see has just been admitted to your maternity unit. The midwife is concerned about her and no other doctor is available to see her at present.

You have 14 minutes to obtain a history from the patient. You seek information relevant to her current pregnancy, determine the reason for her admission and formulate a management plan.

Examination reveals normal vital signs, her urine is normal. On abdominal palpation, the uterus is equivalent to her dates with a breech presentation. On vaginal examination, the cervix is effaced but not dilated, presenting part at the level of spines with intact membranes. An obstetric calculator is supplied.

YOU WILL BE AWARDED MARKS FOR YOUR ABILITY TO:

- Take a history
- Make a diagnosis
- Formulate a management plan

Role-player's instructions

- Disinterested attitude and awkward to the point of being obstructive, but in pain.
- You are 21 years old; this is your second pregnancy, which has reached 29 weeks.
- LMP – date of exam minus 29 weeks, giving appropriate EDD.
- This pregnancy is unplanned, resulting from a casual relationship and failed barrier contraception. Your previous pregnancy was terminated at 8 weeks as you were then 15 years old and still at school.
- You booked at the maternity unit at 16 weeks.
- All the blood tests were normal.
- Antenatal care has been shared with your general practitioner.
- Ultrasound at 18 weeks showed a normally grown fetus equivalent to your dates. The ultrasonographer noted the presence of a choroid plexus cyst. You were seen by the consultant and reassured. Rescan at 24 weeks did not show any choroid plexus cyst.
- The day before admission you had felt generally unwell with crampy abdominal pains. Several hours prior to admission you developed abdominal pains that were intermittent and are now lasting about 30 seconds with 2–3 minutes in between. You have also had some vaginal discharge that is slimy with some bloodstaining.
- Personal – single, unemployed live at home with parents, three brothers and two sisters. You are the eldest.
- Family – mother is a non-identical twin.
- Social – you smoke 20 cigarettes per day, and drink alcohol at the weekends (six to seven bottles of lager), depending on the cash flow situation.
- Drugs – occasional ecstasy tablet but not since you found out you were pregnant. Never used i.v. drugs. Use inhalers (becotide and ventolin) for asthma.
- You ask the candidate, 'What is the cause of the pain?'

Mark sheet

History

Presenting complaint

- Duration of pregnancy
- Contractions – sequence and timing
- 'Show'

Current pregnancy

- Unplanned
- Shared care
- LMP/EDD
- Scan result

Past history

- Obstetric
- Social
- Drugs
- Family
- Medical

0 1 2 3 4 5 6

Provisional diagnosis

- Preterm labour
- Investigate cause
- Infection
- Differential diagnosis urine tract infection (UTI), appendicitis, concealed abruption or bowel problems

0 1 2 3 4 5

Treatment plan

- Admit; discuss aims of treatment to prolong the pregnancy
- Try to stop contractions
- Steroids
- Discuss with paeds
- Mode of delivery

0 1 2 3 4 5

Global score

0 1 2 3 4

Total /20

Circuit B, Station 3

Urinary incontinence

Candidate's instructions

The patient you are about to see was referred to your outpatient clinic by her general practitioner. A copy of the referral letter is given below. You should accept the GP's examination findings as correct.

You have 14 minutes to read the letter and obtain a relevant history from the patient. You should discuss any relevant investigations and treatment that you feel may be indicated with the patient.

Dear Doctor

Please see Mrs Martha Black who is a part-time schoolteacher and who has been experiencing urinary incontinence for 4–5 years.

She can feel a lump coming down and it is affecting her lifestyle.

She is overweight and her current body mass index (BMI) is 32. General physical examination was normal, but she has a moderate cystourethrocele. A recent cervical smear test was normal, and an MSU showed *E. coli*.

Please see and treat as required.

Yours sincerely

Dr Beattie

YOU WILL BE AWARDED MARKS FOR:

- Obtaining a relevant history from the patient
- Discussing relevant investigations
- Discussing appropriate management options

Role-player's instructions

- You are Mrs Martha Black, a 53-year-old woman who works as a part-time schoolteacher. Your main problems are as follows:
  - urinary frequency, passing urine eight to 10 times per day
  - passing urine at night (nocturia) – two to three times per night
  - no bedwetting
  - when you've got to go, you've got to go, with occasional accidents of not getting there on time
  - you leak when you cough, laugh, sneeze and run for a bus, and so do not do much exercise to try to reduce your weight as it is too embarrassing
  - occasional stinging on passing urine.
- You went through the menopause at age 48 years, with no gynaecological problems. You have had three children, all normal deliveries and all weighing over 4 kg. You remain sexually active.
- The rest of the history is unremarkable, although you smoke 20 cigarettes per day and seem to be always 'chesty'.
- You are overweight but claim not to eat very much at all; you drink at least 10 cups of tea/coffee per day and have a cuppa just before going to bed.
- Whenever the doctor suggests investigations, you need to ask exactly what does it involve. Ask about how the bladder pressure studies are performed and why they are done.

Mark sheet

Relevant history

- Basic symptoms, frequency, nocturia, urgency, dysuria
- Incontinence type
- Basic gynaecological history
- Obstetric history, deliveries and size of babies
- Food intake, especially quantity and timing of tea
- Family and social history, including smoking

0 1 2 3 4 5

Relevant investigations

- Repeat MSU to ensure it has been treated
- Random blood sugar, or possibly a fasting one
- Urodynamics – needs to explain what is done with a catheter in the bladder, transducer in the rectum and filling the bladder and looking at the voiding. Not dignified but not painful. Need to ensure MSU negative before undertaking it

0 1 2 3 4 5

Management options

- Recommend weight loss and stopping smoking
- Refer for physiotherapy and pelvic floor exercises
- May benefit from HRT
- Treat UTI if still present
- May need to manage non-insulin-dependent diabetes if indicated by blood glucose levels
- Reduce fluid intake, especially caffeine intake. Advice on timing of intake to reduce nocturia. May be useful to keep a fluid diary for a few days to get the message home
- See in 3 months for review

0 1 2 3 4 5 6

Global score

0 1 2 3 4

Total /20

Circuit B, Station 4

Urinary incontinence viva

Candidate's instructions

You are about to discuss the further management of the patient who you saw in the previous station. The examiner will ask you a number of questions relating to this further management

The plan of management should have been as follows:

- Recommend weight loss and stop smoking
- Refer for physiotherapy and pelvic floor exercises
- May benefit from HRT
- Treat UTI
- Reduce fluid intake
- See in 3 months for review.

She now attends 3 months later and there is no appreciable change in her symptoms. She feels that the lump in her vagina has been getting worse.

The results of her investigations are as follows:

- MSU – negative
- Blood sugar normal
- Urodynamics showed a normal cystometric capacity, minimal residual volume, good flow rate. Stable bladder with genuine stress incontinence demonstrated.

The examiner will also ask you four specific questions relating to her further management during the next 14 minutes.

YOU WILL BE MARKED ON YOUR ABILITY TO ANSWER THE QUESTIONS REGARDING SURGICAL MANAGEMENT

Examiner's instructions

At this station, the candidate will have 14 minutes to discuss the further management of the patient seen earlier (in Station 3). Familiarize yourself with the candidate's instructions. You should ask the candidates the following questions:

What surgical operations are open to this patient and what are their basic differences?

- Anterior repair ± hysterectomy
- Transvaginal tape (TVT)
- Colposuspension
- Needle suspension Stamey/Raz
- Sling procedures – not appropriate as first line
- ?Sacrocolpopexy
- Injectable agents

Discusses the differences between the suprapubic approach, vaginal approach and procedures for failure of initial procedures.

0 1 2 3 4

What are the objective success rates of these surgical procedures?

- Success would be continence or a substantial improvement
- Anterior repair: 1 year < 70 per cent; 5 years < 40 per cent
- TVT: 1 year 80+ per cent, long-term studies ongoing
- Colposuspension: 1 year 90 per cent; 20 year up to 70 per cent
- Stamey: 1 year 80–90 per cent; 5 years 60–70 per cent
- Sling operation not appropriate as first operation in this case

0 1 2 3 4

What are the possible intraoperative and postoperative complications and how these problems would be managed?

- Bleeding, pressure, diathermy or in a colposuspension continuing to tie the support sutures
- Bladder damage, use of dye in the bladder
- Infection – preoperative antibiotics
- Retention of urine postoperatively, suprapubic catheter
- Detrusor instability (10 per cent)
- Enterocele 10–20 per cent
- Sexual problems secondary to vaginal shortening and narrowing

0 1 2 3 4

Describe how you would perform a Burch colposuspension would be undertaken

- Routine preoperative work-up
- GA, TED stockings
- Lloyd Davis position, prepping the skin and towel, urethral catheter, ?methylene blue in bladder
- Suprapubic incision, specify the layers
- Identify cave of Retzius/retropubic space
- Identifying where sutures to be placed, and type (ethibond) and number, from paraurethral tissue to pectineal line
- Closure and insertion of suprapubic catheter and drain
- Writing notes

0 1 2 3 4

Global score

0 1 2 3 4

Total /20

Circuit B, Station 5

Operative – Caesarean section

Candidate's instructions

You are the registrar coming on duty at the time of routine handover. Mrs Jones is in Room 6. She is a primip who has been in labour for 12 hours and over the past 6 hours has remained at 9 cm dilatation despite the use of syntocinon over the past 2 hours. There is one-fifth of the head palpable abdominally on bimanual examination with caput and moulding of the head. The CTG has remained normal throughout, despite a trace of meconium on the pad. A decision has already been made for the patient to have a Caesarean section and you will have to do it.

You are asked to describe in detail:

- the steps required in relation to the decision for LSCS, discussion, consent preparation
- the procedure itself
- the patient's postoperative care and the plan for future pregnancies.

The examiner will ask you a number of questions over the next 14 minutes.

Examiner's instructions

Familiarize yourself with the candidate's instructions. You should ask the candidate to describe in detail the steps required in relation to the decision for LSCS, discussion, consent preparation and the procedure itself, the patient's postoperative care and the plan for future pregnancies.

You will need to cover aspects of the procedure that relate to Caesarean section in general and also the factors that relate to the specific case.

Do not prompt the candidate.

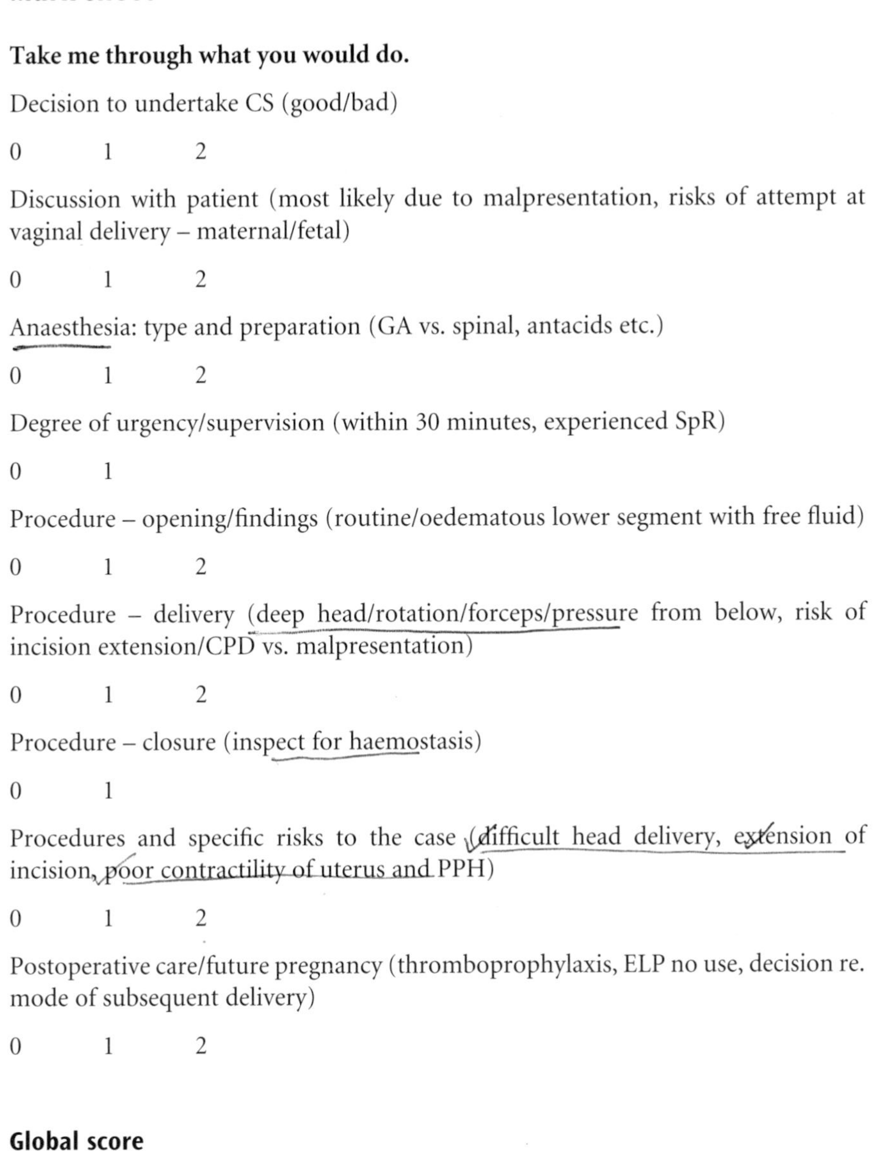

Mark sheet

Take me through what you would do.

Decision to undertake CS (good/bad)

0 1 2

Discussion with patient (most likely due to malpresentation, risks of attempt at vaginal delivery – maternal/fetal)

0 1 2

Anaesthesia: type and preparation (GA vs. spinal, antacids etc.)

0 1 2

Degree of urgency/supervision (within 30 minutes, experienced SpR)

0 1

Procedure – opening/findings (routine/oedematous lower segment with free fluid)

0 1 2

Procedure – delivery (deep head/rotation/forceps/pressure from below, risk of incision extension/CPD vs. malpresentation)

0 1 2

Procedure – closure (inspect for haemostasis)

0 1

Procedures and specific risks to the case (difficult head delivery, extension of incision, poor contractility of uterus and PPH)

0 1 2

Postoperative care/future pregnancy (thromboprophylaxis, ELP no use, decision re. mode of subsequent delivery)

0 1 2

Global score

0 1 2 3 4

Total **/20**

Circuit B, Station 6 ✓

Abnormal smear

Candidate's instructions

The general practitioner has referred the patient you are about to see to your colposcopy clinic. A copy of the referral letter is given below. Read the letter and obtain a relevant history from the patient. You should discuss any relevant investigations and treatment that you feel may be indicated.

The Surgery
High Rd
Buckhurst Hill

Dear Doctor

Re: Mrs Joan Starr (23.10.74)

I would be pleased if you could see this patient whose recent cervical smear result showed severe dyskaryosis with wart viral infection.

She is nulliparous and the rest of her medical history is unremarkable.

Yours sincerely

Dr S. White

MARKS WILL BE AWARDED FOR:
- Relevant history-taking
- Explaining result
- Discussion of relevant treatment options

You have 14 minutes.

Role-player's instructions

You are Joan Sturr, a 30-year-old woman who works as a secretary. You have been completely freaked out by your abnormal smear result and have two things on your mind:

- You think this result means that you have got cancer.
- Your partner (husband) has been unfaithful and has given you the wart virus, and this is entirely his fault.

You are completely asymptomatic; you have never been pregnant and have never had any sexually transmitted diseases. You have only ever had three sexual partners and do not really like talking about sexual matters. You are, however, taking the pill but no other medication and have no other medical history of note. You smoke 20 cigarettes per day but this has recently increased since discovering the smear result.

You are anxious to know more about the procedure of colposcopy: will it hurt and how long will it take for the results? You want to know the treatment options and might consider alternative therapies because you are afraid of hospitals. Your mother died from breast cancer at the age of 54 years. You are also anxious about your fertility as you were planning to stop the pill to try for a pregnancy and only had the smear taken to check all was well before doing so. This is your first smear.

Examiner's instructions

At this station, the candidate will have 14 minutes to obtain a history relevant to the patient's complaint. The candidate should also discuss with the patient what colposcopy entails and that a biopsy may be necessary.

The candidate needs to explain to the patient that cytology is looking for a premalignant lesion, and to sensibly explain what the term 'wart virus infection' means.

Mark sheet

History

- Symptoms IMB/PCB
- Basic gynaecological history/contraception
- Obstetric history
- Genital tract infections
- Family and social history, including smoking
- Allergies, especially to iodine and peanut oil if sultrin cream to be used

0 1 2 3 4 5 6

Colposcopy counselling

- Explains what happens – looking at the transformation zone and why
- Biopsy needed
- Usually gives a good idea of what is going on by the end of the procedure
- Explains that the screening programme is looking for premalignant disease
- This smear result is suggestive of precancer
- More than likely needs treatment
- Avoids blaming any particular partner

0 1 2 3 4 5

Treatment

- Advises stopping smoking and why
- Explains about LLTZ and that it could be done as an outpatient or GA
- Could see and treat at this procedure but would depend on colposcopic findings
- Need for follow-up after treatment
- At some point explains that this should not affect her fertility

0 1 2 3 4 5

Global score

0 1 2 3 4

Total: /20

Circuit B, Station 7

CTG abnormality

You are called to see Mrs Dunne in Room 4. She is a 22-year-old primip who is now term + 7 days in an otherwise uneventful first pregnancy. She was booked for induction of labour in 4 days' time. She has presented with some irregular contractions, decreased fetal movements and a show. The midwife is worried about the CTG which she shows you.

You are asked to counsel the patient and her partner about the management of the labour. Her vital signs are normal. The cervix is 2 cm dilated but fully effaced and the head is 2 cm above the spines.

MARKS WILL BE AWARDED FOR:

- Discussing the CTG
- Discussing further management of this labour

You have 14 minutes at this station.

Role-player's brief

You are 22 years old and you live with your partner who works for Greenpeace. You had initially wanted a home birth with as little intervention as possible. You have been well throughout the pregnancy and noticed some tightenings during the night with a show and slight decrease in the baby's movements. You are convinced it is a girl and keep calling her Flora.

Your partner is devoted to you and you are constantly looking to him for support. You are reluctant to be monitored and do so grudgingly for Flora's sake, but feel that the whole of the medical profession is male-dominated and wants to do Caesarean sections on everyone.

You are concerned about the welfare of your baby and want the registrar to be very explicit about why he is worried about the trace. If he does not pick up on the severity of the trace, you need to get him to explain why it doesn't look like the one in your pregnancy book.

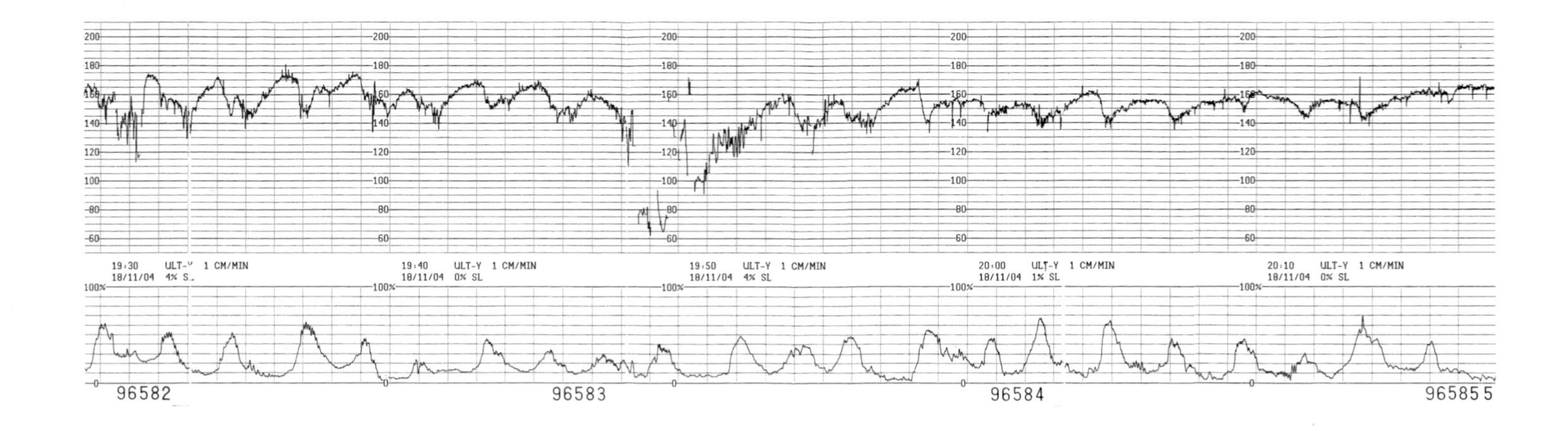
19:30 ULT-Y 1 CM/MIN
18/11/04 4% S.
19:40 ULT-Y 1 CM/MIN
18/11/04 0% SL
19:50 ULT-Y 1 CM/MIN
18/11/04 4% SL
20:00 ULT-Y 1 CM/MIN
18/11/04 1% SL
20:10 ULT-Y 1 CM/MIN
18/11/04 0% SL
96582
96583
96584
965855

Mark sheet

Discusses CTG under broad headings

- Define risk, decreased fetal movements and past due date
- Contraction regularity
- Baseline rate – tachycardia
- Variability – reduced
- Accelerations – none
- Decelerations – shallow
- Opinion – non-reassuring/abnormal

0 1 2 3 4 5 6 7

Concern about status of baby

- Early stage of labour
- Unable to do FBS
- Possible diagnosis of abruptio or feto-maternal transfusion

0 1 2 3 4

Discusses LSCS

- Type of anaesthesia (spinal vs. GA), allows partner to be present
- Consent
- Portrays the urgency of the situation

0 1 2 3 4 5

Global score

0 1 2 3 4

Total: /20

Circuit B, Station 8

Down's syndrome

Candidate's instructions

Ms Cropper, aged 40 years, and her partner have come to the antenatal clinic to discuss their Down's syndrome screening and CVS results. They had expected to see the consultant but he has been called away and you are left to counsel this couple who have been waiting at least 1 hour. At this station you are asked to counsel the couple and discuss the further management of this pregnancy.

The results of the quadruple test and the subsequent scan and chorionic villous sampling are as follows:

Neural tube defect and Down's syndrome screening (Ms CROPPER, aged 40)
SCREEN POSITIVE at 16 weeks' gestation
Increased risk of Down's syndrome of 1 in 50 (background risk 1 in 100)

Anomaly scan at 17 weeks
No obvious fetal anomalies

CVS result
Abnormal – trisomy 21

YOU WILL BE AWARDED MARKS FOR:

- Explaining the diagnosis and implications
- Further management and appropriate counselling

Role-player's instructions

You are a professional unmarried couple and this is your first pregnancy. Ms Cropper is a 40-year-old teacher. You had expected to see the consultant to discuss the Down's syndrome screening and are disgruntled at the length of wait and the apparently casual attitude of the staff you have come across to date. You eventually get to see the registrar (the candidate) who should introduce himself/herself. If not, ask the candidate exactly who they are and what is their level of experience.

You are not convinced of the result as the couple who had the chorionic villous sampling before you looked 'far more likely to have a Down's syndrome baby than us' (your words) – could the results have been mixed up?

The candidate should explore the results with you and the reason for having the screening in the first place, i.e. your age risk. All the results point to the diagnosis being correct. The options that you want to discuss are termination and what it involves, and the possibility of continuing the pregnancy. The candidate should offer to arrange a paediatric consultation for you but you should not lead the candidate in this particular area.

You are naturally upset and concerned about the possibility of future pregnancies and how, if you have a termination, you are going to cope with it mentally and how much time will you need off work.

Mark sheet

- Explains diagnosis
- Apologizes for delay
- Explains the results, avoiding jargon
- Answers questions sensitively and without interrupting

0 1 2 3 4 5 6

Further management

- Explains the reason for the test in the first place was age-related
- Offers options of termination or continuing pregnancy
- If continuing pregnancy, offers paediatric consultation
- Explains termination
  - cervagem
  - mifepristone
  - extra-amniotic
  - risk of ERPC
  - postmortem may be useful

0 1 2 3 4 5

Appropriate counselling

- Gives them option to come back after a time to think it over
- Counselling after TOP before and after
- Follow-up and trying for another pregnancy

0 1 2 3 4 5

Global score

0 1 2 3 4

Total: /20

Circuit B, Station 9

Ectopic pregnancy – explain laparoscopy

Candidate's instructions

The casualty officer initially referred the patient you are about to see. You have already seen Angela Benham (who is a Jehovah's Witness) in the accident and emergency department with vaginal spotting and severe left iliac fossa pain, which had been present for 6 hours. She is otherwise fit and well. She has had unprotected intercourse and her last menstrual period was 7 weeks ago. You suspected an ectopic pregnancy. The pregnancy test is positive and the ultrasound scan now shows an empty uterus.

You feel she needs a laparoscopy in the first instance. Explain the suspected diagnosis and the proposed management to Ms Benham.

MARKS WILL BE AWARDED FOR:

- Explaining the diagnosis
- Discussing treatment options
- Identifying and answering patient's concerns

You have 14 minutes.

Role-player's instructions

You are Angela Benham, a 28-year-old woman who works as a personal assistant. You have been trying to get pregnant over the past 6–12 months. You have presented with some vaginal bleeding and quite severe pain in the left lower quadrant of your abdomen. You have already done a home pregnancy test, which was positive. You have had a vaginal scan, which was uncomfortable, and are waiting for the registrar to talk to you about the results.

He/she is going to tell you that the pregnancy is in the tube and that you will need a laparoscopy (telescope) into the abdomen and may need some other form of surgery. You have no idea about your reproductive anatomy and must get him to explain in layman's terms. As he continues you realize that you have lost the pregnancy whatever happens and you get very emotional about it. You are also worried about future fertility and contraception.

You are a Jehovah's Witness and are adamant about no blood products.

Questions you may ask

- 'Why is it not in the uterus?'
- 'Can't it be moved into the uterus?'
- 'Can I go and see my GP to discuss it'
- 'I need to talk to my husband'
- Are there any drugs that can be used to salvage the pregnancy?'
- Ask about future fertility, as you have been trying for 6–12 months to get pregnant
- 'What are the risks of it happening again?'
- 'I don't want a hysterectomy'
- 'Are you going to kill my baby and what is going to happen to it?'
- 'Are you telling me I am going to have an abortion?'

Mark sheet

- Explains the diagnosis of tubal pregnancy correctly, i.e. 7 weeks amenorrhoea, positive pregnancy test and empty uterus on scan
- Acknowledges pregnancy loss/bereavement aspect

0 1 2 3 4

Management

- Explains urgency of the situation
- Explains proposed management laparoscopy (possible laparotomy)
- Explains salpingostomy/salpingectomy (RCOG guidelines)
- Explains the procedures of the above

0 1 2 3 4

Discusses future fertility

- Ovarian function
- Risk of a further ectopic
- Discusses future types of contraception

0 1 2 3 4

Deals with JW aspect

- Talks about the possibility of large blood loss
- Needs to test for blood group and risk of isoimmunization
- Possible autotransfusion
- Discusses patient signing a separate consent form

0 1 2 3 4

Global score

0 1 2 3 4

Total: /20

Circuit B, Station 10

Breech delivery

Candidate's instructions

Delivery unit emergency call

Doctor, please come to Room 6 immediately, Mrs Pearson gravida 4, para 3 under the care of an independent midwife is in advanced labour with an undiagnosed breech presentation.

You are asked to discuss with the examiner how you would proceed and will then be asked a number of questions pertinent to the case. A doll and mannequin are available for you to take the examiner through a breech delivery.

YOU WILL BE AWARDED MARKS FOR:

- Dealing appropriately with the situation
- Conduct of the breech delivery
- Subsequent examiner's questions

You have 14 minutes.

Examiner's instructions

Ask the candidate: 'Take me through what you would do?'

Prompt

'Would you like any other information?'

Information available

- Normal pregnancy
- Normal obstetric history
  - SVD: 3.4 kg
  - SVD: 3.6 kg
  - SVD: 3.6 kg
- Term
- SRM 2 hours previously, no meconium
- Observations normal, FHR 150 bpm, intermittent auscultation
- VE – fully dilated
- Breech RSL distending introitus with contractions
- Doll and pelvis present for the candidate to take examiner through breech delivery.

Once the candidate has finished the delivery, the following questions should be asked:

- 'What is the role of ECV in this case and generally?'
- 'What are the contraindications to ECV?'
- 'How would you have managed this patient had you seen her the week prior to delivery?'

Mark sheet

Asks appropriate history:

- Weight of previous babies.
- Current gestation and any problems
- When did the membranes rupture
- The colour of liquor
- Has monitoring been normal so far

0 1 2 3 4

Examines abdomen to assess:

- Size of baby
- Descent of presenting part
- Asks for vaginal findings and suggests that he/she confirm them

0 1 2 3

Conduct of Breech Delivery:

- Places thumbs and fingers appropriately on fetal spine and iliac crest
- Avoids touching the baby's abdomen
- Does not use traction, but guides baby
- Keeps sacrum and back anterior (uppermost), made need to hold baby to avoid rotation
- Allows time for body to hang
- Delivers head appropriately, either forceps to after coming head, or Mauriceau-Smellie-Veit manoeuvre. Avoids pulling on the jaw and understands the importance of keeping head flexed with malar pressure

0 1 2 3 4 5 6

Answers questions appropriately:

0 1 2 3

Global score

0 1 2 3 4

Total score /20

Circuit C

Circuit C, Station 1

Vicar's daughter – ethics

Candidate's instructions

You are doing a regular session in the family planning clinic while taking some time off full-time employment to study for the MRCOG. Last month Jocelyn Broody, the local vicar's only child, came to see you for some contraception advice. She wanted you to prescribe the pill for her, as her relationship with her boyfriend has become sexually intimate. Although you encourage her to use a barrier method, and by the end of the consultation you are happy to prescribe the pill for her, Jocelyn is 15 years old. She does not want her parents to know.

The next person on your list today is one of Jocelyn's parents, who is the person in front of you. You suspect rightly that the reason for the appointment is that Jocelyn's parent has found out and wishes to question the morality of your action and its legality.

MARKS WILL BE AWARDED FOR:

- Dealing with a difficult situation
- Explaining the ethical issues

You have 14 minutes.

Role-player's instructions

You have discovered that Jocelyn, just 15 years old, and your only child, is on the pill, which you found whilst tidying her bedroom in her absence. You know that she goes out with a group of her friends, but you were not aware that she was intimately involved with anyone in particular.

You are the local vicar's wife and do not approve of extramarital relationships. You think that whoever prescribed the pill was acting unlawfully in that:

- you as her parent should have been consulted
- given that it is a criminal offence to have sex with someone under 16 years, the doctor is an accessory to a crime.

You suspect rightly that this family planning doctor prescribed the pill for Jocelyn and you decide to confront the doctor with your findings and complain mainly about two issues:

- why you weren't consulted
- the legality of what the doctor has done, as Jocelyn is only 15.

When the doctor talks about Jocelyn's competency, you ask how she can be assessed as competent when she is only 15 years old. You close the scenario by saying that you have heard the advice/explanations given; that you want to share them with your husband and perhaps arrange to come again as a couple.

Examiner's instructions

The purpose of this station is for the candidate to diffuse a potentially irate parent. The doctor has acted within the law and has acted in the patient's (the daughter's) interest. There is a confidentiality issue in not disclosing information to the mother despite the daughter being under the age of consent.

Ethical issues covered

- Acting in the best interest of the child
- Not prepared to divulge contents of Jocelyn's consultation
- Mother may want to consider TOP option if no contraception
- Non-judgmental in attitudes and behaviour
- Duty of care is to the patient and not to the relative
- Need to be aware of Data Protection Act, which does not allow disclosure of patient information

0 1 2 3 4 5

Following 'illegality prompt'

- Not illegal to prescribe contraceptive to under-16s
- Mention the House of Lords decision in Gillick case/Fraser guidelines

0 1 2 3

Assessment of Gillick competency/Fraser guidelines

- Should discuss this generally and avoid mentioning the daughter.
- Assesses the ability of a 15 year old girl to understand what is going on, the consequences and risks
- A girl in this situation is encouraged to inform her parents, and the reasons for not doing so are usually explored
- A girl is informed that her confidentiality would be respected
- A doctor can consider that a girl, if competent, can consent to examination and treatment under 16 years of age

0 1 2 3 4 5

Follow-up

- Offers to meet mother ± father with the daughter, but would only talk about medical problems with the daughter's consent and ideally in person. Verbal consent to mother is not adequate
- Is explicit about the confidentiality aspect of the patient/doctor relationship

0 1 2 3

Global score (overall competency)

0 1 2 3 4

Total: /20

Circuit C, Station 2

Shoulder dystocia

Candidate's instructions

Delivery unit emergency call: 'Doctor, please come to Room 4 immediately, as Mrs Pearson, gravida 2, para 1, has delivered the head but the shoulders are stuck.'

You are the doctor called to this delivery. Discuss with the examiner how you would proceed. A doll and mannequin have been provided for you to demonstrate the delivery.

YOU WILL BE MARKED ON YOUR ABILITY TO DEMONSTRATE YOUR PRACTICAL SKILLS

You have 14 minutes.

Examiner's instructions

Say to the candidate: 'Take me through what you would do, and how you would deliver.' You should ask the candidate to deliver the doll.

After the candidate has finished, ask the following questions:

- at what speed does the cord pH drop?
- what are the predisposing factors to shoulder dystocia?
- what is occurrence of shoulder dystocia in normal weight babies?
- how would you repair the third-degree tear?

Mark sheet

Management of shoulder dystocia

H	Call for help, anaesthetist, paediatrician
E	Evaluate for episiotomy and extend if possible
L	Legs McRoberts manoeuvre (hyperflexion of the hips)
P	Pressure, external pressure, understanding of the direction of pressure, i.e. the posterior aspect of the shoulder
E	Enter Wood's Screw Manoeuvre
R	Rotate posterior shoulder to anterior
R	Roll over onto all fours

Continue each for 30 seconds before moving onto the manoeuvre. Understands the importance of moving the shoulder anteriorly across the abdomen to narrow the diameter. Pushing it in the opposite direction increases the diameter.

0 1 2 3 4 5 6 7 8 9

After the candidate has finished, the following should be asked:

- The speed at which the cord pH drops
- The predisposing factors to shoulder dystocia
- Occurrence in normal weight babies
  - The cord pH falls 0.04 per minute
  - 50% occur with a normal weight
  - Predisposing factors GDM, raised BMI of mother, large baby, postmaturity

0 1 2 3

- How do you repair the third degree tear and what postoperative management do you advise?
  - Describes overlap method or end-to-end (no reliable evidence to show that either is superior)
  - Preferably do repair in operating theatre under regional or general anaesthesia
  - PDS is superior to catgut or polyglactin as it is associated with less infection and better long-term function of the anal sphincter complex. (Catgut no longer on UK market)
  - Broad spectrum antibiotics should be given intra-operatively and post-operatively
  - Post-operative laxatives are associated with less post-operative wound dehiscence
  - Risk management form and needs postnatal follow-up appointment
  - All women with a third degree tear should be seen at 6–12 months by a

gynaecologist with an interest in anal-rectal dysfunction or a colorectal surgeon

0 1 2 3 4

Global score

0 1 2 3 4

Total Score: /20

Circuit C, Station 3

Breaking bad news – ovarian cancer

Candidate's instructions

The next patient has been sent down from the general surgical ward to your 'fast-track' clinic. She is Mrs Julie Dunlop, aged 45 years, and she was originally referred with a history of dyspepsia, flatulence, some weight loss and a slightly bloated abdomen. She was admitted via A&E with abdominal pain. On rectal examination she was found to have a mass in the pelvis.

An ultrasound scan of the abdomen and pelvis shows a complex mass 8 cm in diameter in the pelvis consistent with a lesion arising from the left ovary. There is a fair degree of free fluid, presumably ascites. A chest X-ray is normal. The CA125 level is 890, and the rest of her blood tests are normal. A CT scan is due to be performed after the clinic visit.

The most likely diagnosis is that of ovarian carcinoma until proved otherwise. Mrs Dunlop is not aware of this tentative diagnosis and has been told that she 'has a cyst that the gynaecology people will sort out for you'.

Your remit is to tell her the most likely diagnosis and outline her further management.

MARKS WILL BE AWARDED FOR:

- Explanation of the possible diagnosis
- Treatment of this presumptive diagnosis

You have 14 minutes.

Role-player's instructions

You are Mrs Julie Dunlop, a 45-year-old housewife with two children aged 12 and 14 years. You have been feeling run-down but felt that it was due to some sleepless nights with your 14-year-old. You have noticed some heartburn and increase in flatulence. You feel that you may have lost weight but your jeans and skirts seem tighter.

You initially thought you might have an ulcer and so were referred to the surgeons. The diagnosis as far as you are concerned is that of an ovarian cyst. The idea of cancer had never entered your head. You become panic-stricken at the thought of what is going to happen to your children.

You keep asking whether the doctor is sure of the diagnosis, and aren't there tablets one can take. You are very apprehensive about surgery. You also mention that you knew someone in the street who had ovarian cancer and she was dead by the Christmas when her operation was in September.

When the doctor mentions chemotherapy, you keep asking whether you are going to lose your hair. You may at this stage ask about your outlook and you may be very specific about life expectancy.

Mark sheet

Explains the diagnosis is possible ovarian cancer

- Explains the scan report
- The significance of the CA125 – sensitive but not always specific
- Avoids non-medical language and emphasizes keeping the patient informed
- Acknowledges the difficulty of taking in the information
- Explains that the good news is that something can be done and discusses outlook realistically
- Treatment would be undertaken in a gynaecological cancer centre – mention cancer centre and unit
- May discuss a differential diagnosis, including endometriosis, fibroma or a possible tumour elsewhere
- Allows patient to ask questions

0 1 2 3 4 5 6 7

May need more imaging CT scan abdominal/pelvis and chest X-rays.

Treatment

- Explains surgery, TAH, BSO and omentectomy, appendicectomy
- Treat as though this were cancer
- Type of incision – midline
- Warns re: catheter, drains, bowel prep, possible NG tube, thromboprophylaxis, lower midline incision, the staging is done at laparotomy, length of stay

0 1 2 3 4 5 6

Discusses chemotherapy

- General overview of adjuvant chemotherapy
- Outlines number of courses and timing – 6 courses, 3 weeks apart at cancer centre

0 1 2 3

Global score

0 1 2 3 4

Total: /20

Circuit C, Station 4

Uterine perforation

Candidate's instructions

The patient you are about to see is postoperative on the gynaecology ward. Kirsty Hadfield was admitted as an emergency last night with a history of 6 weeks' bleeding following a normal delivery. Her Hb was 9.8 g%. An ultrasound scan was performed which suggested the presence of an echogenic area in the uterine cavity. It was decided that she needed an evacuation of the uterus.

She was taken to theatre and an evacuation was performed. Unfortunately, during this procedure the uterus was perforated and bowel was pulled through the cervix. This was when you were called to theatre. You undertook a laparoscopy, which showed a perforation and bleeding, so you proceeded to a laparotomy. You oversewed the perforation, which was adjacent to a few small fibroids, and you wondered whether there could have been some degeneration of one of them to make the uterus so soft and consequently more susceptible to perforation. The rest of the pelvis looks normal. The sigmoid looked all right and only required oversewing of the serosal surface.

You have come to explain the findings to the patient and their implications for the future.

YOU WILL BE AWARDED MARKS FOR:
- Explaining the operative findings
- Future implications and management
- Dealing with her concerns

You have 14 minutes.

Role-player's instructions

You are Kirsty Hadfield, a 28-year-old woman who works as a legal secretary. You delivered 6 weeks ago and have continued to bleed vaginally ever since. You have been fobbed off a few times by your GP with courses of antibiotics but have finally been admitted.

You signed a consent form for evacuation of the uterus (D&C) but now have pain in your abdomen and have pressure dressing over a wound. There is a drain and urinary catheter in place. You are concerned that they have taken away the uterus.

Questions you may ask

- 'What did you do, did you do a hysterectomy?'
- 'Why did this happen?'
- 'What happens if I try for another baby?'
- 'Did the fibroids have anything to do with it?'
- 'Why didn't you remove the fibroids?'
- 'Is this because people have fobbed me off with antibiotics?'
- 'I want to see the consultant' – become increasingly bolshie about having been operated on by a junior member of the staff and this happening.
- 'Why didn't you wake me up and discuss it?'

Mark sheet

Explains the operative findings and procedures performed

- Explains laparoscopy bleeding
- Explains concerns at evacuation of uterus
- Discusses the possibility of uterine perforation being due to infection or degeneration of the fibroids
- Allows questions along the way
- Tries to be open and non-defensive
- Deals with bowel injury

0 1 2 3 4 5 6

Discusses future fertility

- Rest of pelvis normal
- Would need to consider mode of delivery at 37 weeks
- More than likely normal delivery
- Discusses future types of contraception

0 1 2 3 4 5

Other concerns

- Discusses the management of the fibroids – risks of removing them at that time may have caused unnecessary bleeding
- May disappear – could scan in 2–3 months' time
- Favours conservative approach unless they become symptomatic
- Will need antibiotics
- Uterus was well emptied at end of procedure

0 1 2 3 4 5

Global score

0 1 2 3 4

Total: /20

Circuit C, Station 5

Postpartum haemorrhage – collapse

Candidate's instructions

Delivery unit emergency call: 'Doctor, please come to Room 6 immediately, Mrs Abbott, gravida 3, para 2, under the care of an independent midwife delivered 2 hours ago and has suddenly collapsed.'

You are the registrar called to see this patient. You need to discuss with the examiner how you would proceed.

YOU WILL BE MARKED ON YOUR ABILITY TO DESCRIBE HOW YOU WOULD DEAL WITH THIS EMERGENCY

You have 14 minutes.

Examiner's instructions

Familiarize yourself with the candidate's instructions. Say to the candidate: 'Take me through what you would do.'

Prompt

'Would you like any other information?'

Information available

- Normal pregnancy
- Normal obstetric history
  - SVD: 3.4 kg
  - SVD: 3.6 kg
- Recent (2 weeks ago) Hb 11.8 g, blood group O (Rh-+ve)
- Normal vaginal delivery, baby weighed 3.5 kg, physiological third stage and placenta appeared complete
- Observations stable throughout the labour and no analgesia was required
- Patient suddenly felt faint, and passed out
- Patient looks pale, pulse rate 110 bpm, BP 90/60
- Small pv blood loss

What candidate should do

- Introduce self to midwife/patient and partner if appropriate
- Examine abdomen to check fundus and rub up contraction if necessary
- Briefly ask about the history of the pregnancy and labour
- Ask about placenta completeness
- Ensure i.v. line(s) inserted and take bloods for FBC, X-match clotting baseline
- May run in haemacel
- May want to check pulse and BP him/herself
- Vaginal examination expels clot, insert catheter
- Ensure input and output well documented
- Discuss the use of syntocinon and ergometrine, including infusion
- Involve the anaesthetist, may need CVP
- Inform senior staff and take to theatre for EUA
- Discuss the 4 Ts: tone, trauma, tissue, thrombin (clotting)
- Use of Hemabate and its contraindications
- B-Lynch suture tying off blood vessels
- Hysterectomy – if not, risks for future pregnancy
- Postoperative ITU
- Mention Sheehan's syndrome
- Debriefing the patient important
- Overall competency

Mark sheet

Appears to be in control of the situation.

0 1 2

Describes clearly what to do.

0 1 2 3

Logical progression of actions.

0 1 2 3

Initiates basic safety measures.

0 1 2

Suggests main causes and solutions.

0 1 2

Importance of vital signs.

0 1 2

Examination.

0 1 2

Global score

0 1 2 3 4

Total: /20

Circuit C, Station 6

Air travel and pregnancy

Candidate's instructions

The patient you are about to see has been referred to your antenatal clinic by her general practitioner. A copy of the referral letter is given below. Read the letter and obtain a relevant history from the patient, discuss the management of this pregnancy and address any concerns she may have regarding it.

The general examination of this patient is normal for her gestation.

Dear Doctor

Re: Ania Wiesnewski

Please see and book this 30-year-old Polish woman for antenatal care. She has been in the UK for 3 years. She is currently 18 weeks pregnant, which was confirmed by a first trimester ultrasound scan in your early pregnancy assessment unit.

Her first pregnancy ended with a fetal death in utero at 28 weeks in 1998. Her history would appear to be otherwise unremarkable. She is keen to visit her grandmother in Poland for her 80th birthday and would like your advice.

Yours sincerely

Dr Lawrence

MARKS WILL BE AWARDED FOR:
- Obtaining a relevant obstetric history
- Explaining the risk factors for this pregnancy
- Addressing any patient concerns

You have 14 minutes.

Role-player's instructions

- You are a 30-year-old Polish woman who has been in this country for 3 years. You have been married for 7 years and work as a part-time cleaner. Your periods are regular, bleeding for 4–5 days every 28 days. You have never had a cervical smear test.
- You smoke 10 cigarettes per day and drink only at the weekend.
- You have no medical history of note, except that you were in a road traffic accident as a child and seem to remember that you may have had a blood transfusion. You are unaware of your blood group. There is no family history of note.
- This is a planned pregnancy – you had some bleeding in early pregnancy for which you had an ultrasound scan so are sure of your dates. Otherwise, there have been no other problems so far in this pregnancy. You are still worried because of previous problems.
- 1998 – planned pregnancy, did not receive very much in the way of antenatal care. You did not see a doctor until about 28 weeks when you noticed that the baby had not moved for about 12 hours. You went to hospital and the baby was found to be dead on scan. A labour was induced and you delivered a stillborn male infant weighing 2.3 kg after 12 hours. There was no PM. There was not much in the way of explanation at home.
- You are keen to visit your grandmother next month for her 80th birthday and you want to know what advice the doctor would give you regarding airline travel.

Mark sheet

- Relevant obstetric histories
- Acknowledges IUFD and obtains further details
- Recognizes SB weight
- May be a macrosomic or a hydropic baby
- Smear discussed – may do opportunistic smear
- Advice re. smoking and alcohol

0 1 2 3 4 5

- Risk factors for this pregnancy
- Recognizes that the weight of the baby was not normal for 28 weeks
- Discusses the possible causes and appropriate investigations in this pregnancy
- Screen for GDM
- Scan to monitor growth/heart defect
- Checks blood group and possible antibodies
- Viral infections, particularly parvovirus

0 1 2 3 4 5 6

Air travel during pregnancy

- Usually not a risk to a healthy pregnant woman
- International travel all right up to 32–35 weeks; advise patient to carry her own notes with the EDD and appropriate insurance
- Aisle seat over a bulkhead provides most space and a seat over the wing in the midplane region will give the smoothest ride
- Advise to walk every 30 minutes and flex and extend ankles frequently
- Safety belt to be fastened at pelvic level
- Fluids to be taken liberally because of dehydrating effect of low humidity in the aircraft
- Support stockings
- If BP raised, should not go; should have BP checked during the time away

0 1 2 3 4 5

Global score

0 1 2 3 4

Total: /20

Circuit C, Station 7

Risk management

Candidate's instructions

Monitoring the frequency of critical incident (or adverse incident) events is an important part of ensuring a high quality of obstetric practice. Your unit wishes to introduce a scheme, which automatically reports critical/adverse incidents during labour.

DISCUSS WITH THE EXAMINER HOW YOU WOULD DEVELOP AND USE A LIST OF IMPORTANT CRITICAL INCIDENTS OR MARKERS TO MONITOR THE INTRAPARTUM CARE IN YOUR MATERNITY UNIT. HOW WOULD YOU INTRODUCE AND MONITOR ITS IMPLEMENTATION? MARKS WILL BE AWARDED FOR A LOGICAL APPROACH AND EXPLANATION

You have 14 minutes.

Mark sheet

Understands the concept of critical or adverse incidents

- Has a logical approach to the problem, e.g. subcategories/classification system

0 1 2 3 4

Introduction of implementation

- Meeting, report forms, risk manager, complaints/medicolegal department, regular review of forms, audit cycle
- Forms a team – multidisciplinary
- Visit other hospitals to see their setup
- Run training programmes
- All staff to know chain of control
- Cross-check that appropriate reporting is occurring (e.g. computer statistics on incidence correlates with number of forms for each incident)

0 1 2 3 4 5 6 7 8

Critical or adverse incident – examples

The candidate should mention examples from the following list which is not exclusive; others can be included – just need to provide a comprehensive list. We would expect a good candidate, in order to score full marks, to mention at least 10.

- Failed induction of labour
- Excess use of prostaglandin agents
- Excess induction delivery interval > 24 hours
- Excess syntocinon infusion
- Uterine hypertonus – initiation of treatment
- Precipitate labour – 3 cm to full dilation < 2 hours
- Malpresentation in labour
- Prolapsed cord in labour
- Fetal disease
  - not confirmed by fetal pH sampling
  - fetal scalp blood pH < 7.1
  - decision to Caesarean section intervals more than 60 minutes
- Ruptured uterus
- Failed forceps
- Failed vacuum extraction
- Combined forceps and vacuum extraction

- Third- and fourth-degree tears
- Intrapartum blood transfusion
- Haemorrhage – intrapartum or postpartum
- Retained placenta, retained placental tissue
- Hb < 8.0 g or fall of 3 g
- Wound breakdown – perineal or Caesarean section
- Return to theatre
- Maternal admission to ICU
- Unexpected maternal pyrexia
- Trauma to other internal organs
- Fetal outcomes
- Apgar score < 5 at 5 minutes
- Unexpected admission to SCBU
- Cord blood pH < 7.00
- Undiagnosed fetal anomaly
- Perinatal sepsis
- Fetal trauma
- Failed epidural
- Failed to receive pain relief
- Dural tap
- Dural headache
- Conversion to GA
- Staffing problems
- Failed to respond to bleep/unable to contact
- Transfer problems

0 1 2 3 4

Global score

0 1 2 3 4

Total: /20

Circuit C, Station 8

Twin pregnancy

Candidate's instructions

Mrs Jarvis, gravida 2, para 1, books into the antenatal clinic under the care of your consultant. She has had a detailed scan at 20 weeks, which shows that she is expecting twins. She is thrilled about the situation and wants to discuss with you what to expect during the rest of the pregnancy and the possibility of a home birth.

YOU WILL BE MARKED ON YOUR ABILITY TO DISCUSS THE RISKS OF A TWIN PREGNANCY, AND THE PLAN FOR DELIVERY

You have 14 minutes.

Examiner's instructions

Say to the candidate: 'Take me through what you would do in this situation.'

Prompt

'Would you like any other information?'

Information available

- 32-year-old teacher, Caucasian
- Normal pregnancy to date
- Normal obstetric history – SVD 3.4 kg
- PMSH normal, no medication and no allergies
- Detailed scan suggest monozygotic twins with two amniotic sacs, otherwise no abnormality
- Blood tests – O, Rh-positive, Hb 11.0 g
- Rest of tests negative

Mark sheet

Asks for other information without prompt

0 1

Explanation of monozygosity

- Needs to pick up on the monozygosity and its higher risk for the fetuses

0 1

Maternal risks

0 1 2 3

Fetal risks

- Needs to cover minor symptoms due to size of uterus as well as the other risks of discordancy, acute polyhydramnios and twin-to-twin transfusion, hypertension, diabetes, premature labour
- Risks to the babies of premature labour, RDS, hypothermia, hypoglycaemia, jaundice, infection etc.
- Problems if very preterm

0 1 2 3

Intrapartum care

0 1 2 3 4

Postpartum care

0 1 2

Dealing with home delivery situation

0 1 2

Global score

0 1 2 3 4

Total: /20

Circuit C, Station 9

Molar pregnancy – counselling

Candidate's instructions

The patient you are about to see is Mrs Astride, who is 43 years old. She had an evacuation of uterus for what was thought to be a delayed miscarriage about 4 weeks ago. The histology has come back showing a complete hydatidiform mole. She was under your consultant's care 3 years ago when she had a Caesarean section for IUGR and PET; a live male infant was delivered at term. She is very concerned about having another child to provide a sibling for her son.

She is unaware of the histology report. You are asked to break the news to her and its implications. You are asked to discuss her further management.

MARKS WILL BE AWARDED FOR:

- Explanation of the diagnosis
- Implications and further management

You have 14 minutes.

Role-player's instructions

You are a 43-year-old social worker called Mrs Brenda Astride. You have one child who was delivered by Caesarean section 3 years ago because of blood pressure problems. He was a little on the small side and weighed 2.5 kg at term.

You are anxious to provide a brother or sister for him and so further fertility is very important to you.

You have recently had a miscarriage and have an inkling that all was not quite right. The doctor will break the news to you. You want to know why this happened. Is there anything that you did to cause this, or anything you could have done to prevent it? What are the risks of it happening again and is there any chance of a further pregnancy? Would it be worth going for IVF?

Mark sheet

- Acknowledges pregnancy loss/bereavement aspect
- Allows patient time to ask questions

0 1 2

- Explains diagnosis
- Explains the diagnosis of molar pregnancy correctly – 90 per cent have duplication of haploid sperm XX and rest dispermic XY; female nuclear DNA is inactivated
- Avoids jargon

0 1 2 3 4

- Implications and further management
- Further management needs to be discussed
- Registration with trophoblastic service
- Chest X-ray
- Beta-HCG levels, urinary and length of follow-up
- Length of follow-up, and contraceptive advice

0 1 2 3 4 5

Implications for future fertility

- 85 per cent have subsequent normal pregnancy
- 2 per cent risk of second mole, 20 per cent risk of third mole
- Background risk of age re. pregnancy loss
- May want to consider ovum donation

0 1 2 3 4 5

Global score

0 1 2 3 4

Total score: /20

Circuit C, Station 10

Results interpretation

Candidate's instructions

At this station you will be given a number of scenarios with the relevant results.

MARKS WILL BE AWARDED FOR DISCUSSING THE FOLLOWING WITH THE EXAMINER:

- Any further information you would like from the patient
- The results, giving an explanation
- The options for further management

Case 1

Ms Mitchell is 29 years old. She has been referred to your gynaecology outpatient clinic with a history of irregular bleeding over the previous 4 months. She has been taking oral contraception over the past 12 months. She has had one full-term normal delivery. Her last cervical smear test was 2 years ago and was normal. She is a heavy smoker.

Results

Ultrasound scan

- Normal sized anteverted uterus, endometrium 4 mm, and midline not seen
- There are three echogenic areas within the cavity – ?polyps
- Both ovaries multifollicular
- Normal adnexae

Answer

Further information required

- Type of oral contraception – exclude progestogen
- Any problems taking oral contraception?
- Any other medication?
- What is her body mass index?

Explanation of results

- Looks like endometrial polyps

Further management options

- Hysteroscopy/D&C and polypectomy
- Location either outpatient or day case, depending on the patient
- Would mirena IUCD be a better option in view of her being a heavy smoker?

Global score

0 1 2 3 4

Case 2

Miss Hennessey is 18 years old and in the first year of a 3-year degree course at university. She presents with a history of secondary amenorrhoea for 18 months. She is also concerned about hirsutism, particularly on her forearms. Her menarche was at 13 years of age and her periods have always been a little erratic.

Her height is 1.67 m and her weight is 43.8 kg, giving a BMI of 16.3.

Results

- LH – 4.7 IU/L
- FSH – 9.3 IU/L
- Prolactin – 205 mU/L (83–527)
- Testosterone – 1.8 nmol/L (0.5–3.0)
- Cortisol – 424 nmol/L (171–800)
- SHBG – 25 nmol/L (38–103)

Ultrasound scan

- Normal sized anteverted uterus, clear cavity
- Left ovary 22 × 15 mm, right ovary 24 × 14 mm
- Multiple tiny follicles consistent with PCOS
- Free fluid in the pouch of Douglas

Answers

Questions

- Why is her BMI so low?
- What are the patient's expectations?

Explanation

- Most likely diagnosis is PCOS, but her low BMI may be a contributing factor – is there any eating disorder?

Options

- Do nothing
- OCP (Dianette) – clomid may be inappropriate at this time
- Induce a withdrawal bleed with provera, but exclude pregnancy
- Cosmesis for hairiness – e.g. waxing, electrolysis
- Warn of need for contraception
- Does the BMI need investigation – either malabsorption or psychiatric referral?

Global score

0 1 2 3 4

Case 3

Mrs Hutchinson, aged 37 years, returns to your clinic for the results of her fertility investigations. She has a regular cycle and no significant history of note.

Results

- Hysterosalpingogram – normal spill of dye through both tubes
- Day 21 serum progesterone – 72 nmol/L
- Sperm count
  - volume: 1.5 mL
  - count: 8 million/mL
  - motility: 40%
  - progressive motility: 50%
  - abnormal forms within normal limits

Answers

Questions
- Around the sample collection and any delay in getting it to the lab
- Partner's habits re. smoking and marijuana
- Type of job/undergarments/baths/illnesses

Explanation
- Patient's results normal
- Sperm count low, may reflect his health 2 months earlier
- Concern as to whether this is the highest or lowest count

Options
- Repeat sperm count at least once
- Possible need for andrology referral
- Decide what the couple want and discuss accordingly
- IUI husband or donor, IVF/ICSI, adoption
- Depends on the couple's views but need to take age into account

Global score

0 1 2 3 4

Case 4

Mrs Jones, aged 59 years, was admitted last night with a history of postmenopausal bleeding which has been happening over the past 3 years. She was unable to pass urine and has recently had difficulty in doing so. She has recently had an abnormal smear and is awaiting a colposcopy appointment. She has no other health problems or any relevant history. Her blood pressure is 150/80. Abdominal examination was unremarkable but vaginal examination revealed a frozen pelvis.

Results

- Hb – 8.3 g
- WCC – 19.0
- Platelets – 641
- Na – 126
- K – 6.0
- Urea – 38.1
- Creatinine – 820

Answers

Questions
- What was the smear abnormality?
- Does she have any pain?
- When did she pass urine?

Explanation
- Anaemia probably secondary to her PMB but she has renal failure, which needs to be dealt with.

Options
- Needs ultrasound scan to see if she has hydronephrosis
- Needs dialysis followed by insertion of nephrostomy tubes
- Referral to the urologists – need to establish a diagnosis and may need EUA, cystoscopy and sigmoidoscopy
- Most likely to be carcinoma of cervix and then will need radiotherapy

Global score

0 1 2 3 4

Case 5

Mrs Astride, aged 43 years, recently underwent an evacuation of uterus for an incomplete miscarriage. She has had one previous pregnancy complicated with pre-eclampsia. She has had some further bleeding and attends the early pregnancy assessment unit for review 10 days after her evacuation and the results from that time are below.

Results

Histology – products of conception consistent with a complete hydatidiform mole.

Answers

Questions

- How much bleeding is present?
- Is the os still open?
- Has a repeat scan been undertaken and, if so, what does it show?

Explanation

- May have some retained products of conception
- May have an endometritis

Options

- May need repeat suction evacuation
- Needs registration with centre (Charing Cross, Sheffield or Dundee)
- Chest X-ray may be needed
- BHCG levels to be done; serum would be useful
- Advice about contraception and planning for further pregnancies needs to be addressed

Global score

0 1 2 3 4

Case 6

Mrs Brough is a 44-year-old woman with a 3-month history of amenorrhoea. She has had one early miscarriage and one full-term normal delivery. Her current BMI is 25. She is not currently using any contraception.

Results

- Serum oestradiol – < 20 pmol/L
- FSH – 69.4 IU/L
- Prolactin – 238 mU/L

Answers

Questions
- Any hot flushes and night sweats?
- Any other symptoms?
- Could she be pregnant and has a pregnancy test been done?

Explanation
- May be climacteric but caution in view of age.

Options
- Repeat FSH 3 months in view of age
- Treat symptomatically with HRT
- Would need contraceptive advice in view of age

Global score

0 1 2 3 4

Case 7

A 35-year-old woman presents with a long-standing history of painful periods but the cycle is regular: 7 days' loss every 28 days. She has had a previous loop cone biopsy for CIN2. On examination, the uterus is clinically 16 weeks size.

Results

Hb – 9.7 g

Ultrasound scan
An enlarged anteverted uterus with multiple small fibroids, the largest being 3–4 cm in diameter. The ovaries look normal.

Answers

Questions
- Any clots or flooding?
- What is her fertility expectation?
- What is her sickle status?
- Any previous treatment?

Explanation
- The haemoglobin level is probably a reflection of chronic blood loss
- Most likely secondary to the fibroids

Options
- Depends on her fertility status and what has been tried before
- Needs oral iron
- Hormonal or non-hormonal treatment, possibly mirena
- Surgery, myomectomy or hysterectomy
- May be a candidate for embolization

Global score

0 1 2 3 4

Mark scored	0–1	2	3	4	5–6	7	8–9	10	11	12–13	14
Mark /20	0	1	2	3	4	5	6	7	8	9	10
Mark scored	15–16	17	18	19–20	21	22–23	24	25	26–27	28	
Mark /20	11	12	13	14	15	16	17	18	19	20	

Index

INDEX